Ancestors, Descendants and Allied Lines
of
Dr. Jacob George Bruckman
1800–1885
and
Dr. Philip Bruckman
1797–1874

German Jewish Immigrant Physicians and Brothers
from Böhmen, Austria (Now Czech Republic)

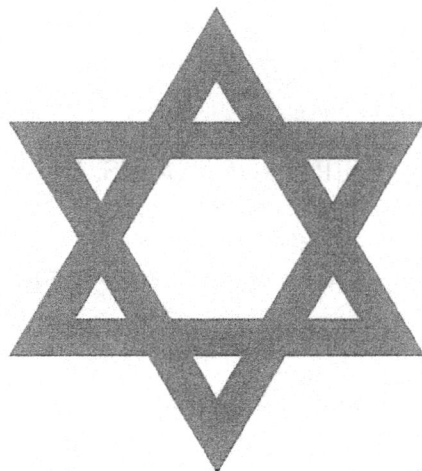

רופא

Compiled and Edited by
Raymond C. Lantz

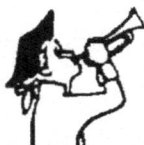

HERITAGE BOOKS
2015

HERITAGE BOOKS
AN IMPRINT OF HERITAGE BOOKS, INC.

Books, CDs, and more—Worldwide

For our listing of thousands of titles see our website
at
www.HeritageBooks.com

Published 2015 by
HERITAGE BOOKS, INC.
Publishing Division
5810 Ruatan Street
Berwyn Heights, Md. 20740

International Standard Book Numbers
Paperbound: 978-0-7884-5675-6
Clothbound: 978-0-7884-6254-2

Preface

This book attempts to document all the known descendants of a Bruckman family who are of German Jewish origins. These Bruckmans trace their origins back to two well known original Jewish settlements known in German as Loschitz and Kremsier. The origins of these Jewish settlements trace back to Roman times, but are most known from the time they became part of the Moravia Provence of the Austrian Empire until their present day inclusion in the Czech Republic.

The reason the author chose to write and compile this Bruckman genealogical work is to inform the many known descendants of their heritage and family origins. The author has devoted more than thirty years of painstaking fruitless research efforts to discover the origins of his branch of this Bruckman family, only to discover in recent months that the key to research success was impeded by unknown hidden family religious backgrounds, believed to have been purposely suppressed to some degree from inclusion in inherited family traditions. For unknown reasons it is blatantly clear that the author's American branch of this family ceased to practice their Jewish faith and did not readily proclaim their previous adherence to same. However, it is through the discovery that one of the first American born members of this branch must have learned from his immigrant father of their Jewish heritage. It is through the author's discovery that this descendent for a period of time in the later 1800's made concerted efforts to maintain periodic personal contact with his immigrant uncle's family. This uncle and his family lived too considerable a distance away for the nephew to be expected to undertake such travel given the period of time in history. Most important is the notoriety of the immigrant uncle and his family with regard to his religious practices and affiliations. They were a very well known and staunch German Jewish immigrant family of New York City.

Once the author ascertained and confirmed that his branch of the Bruckman family was in fact German Jewish, this provided the missing research key that led the author and others on a fast and furious, as well as extremely fruitful, research journey. This journey very quickly uncovered the true origins of this Bruckman family that had escaped the author and many other descendants and researchers for many decades, approaching nearly a century in research time.

For the above stated reasons it gives the author great pleasure and satisfaction to provide the information relating to the heritage and origins of the Bruckman family contained herein. As well as being able to clearly identify as many descendant lines as currently possible given the current research sources readily available to the author.

Raymond Clyde Lantz

Acknowledgment

The author wishes to extend his many thanks and eternal gratitude to all the fellow researchers and cousins who willingly shared and exchanged information throughout the many years regarding our common ancestors. Special thanks goes out to the author's cousin William "Bill" Richard Griffin, whose personal contact and initiative provided critical information that led to the successful research of the origins of our Bruckman ancestors. Without this initial family historical information passed down to him and shared with the author, the creation of this book and the family information it contains would not have been possible.

Table of Contents

HOW TO USE THIS BOOK

In Chapter 1 the oldest known Bruckman and every direct descendant is given a unique alpha or alpha numeric identification ID. The oldest known person in Generation 1 is identified as Roman numeral "I".

All the known children of Generation 1 or Generation 2 are identified beginning with Roman numeral "II" and subsequent.

All the known children of Generation 2 or Generation 3 are identified beginning with the alphabet letter "A" and subsequent.

Chapters 2 through 6 are each devoted to one of the known Generation 3 descendants and all of their known descendants. Each successive generation descendant is identified by adding a sequential number or letter to the end of the parent descendant's ID to create a new unique descendant ID.

The following example illustrates the lineal descent of the author as contained in Chapter 6 of this book:

I LAZARAS BRUCKMAN (Gen 1)

    II MOSHE BRUCKMAN I (Gen 2)

        E JACOB GEORGE BRUCKMAN II (Gen 3)

            E3 FRANKLIN DAVID BRUCKMAN E (Gen 4)

                E35 CHARLES HERBERT BRUCKMAN E3 (Gen 5)

                    E355 DORIS FAYE BRUCKMAN E35 (Gen 6)

                        E3551 RAYMOND CLYDE LANTZ E355 (Gen 7)

Once a known descendant is located in the book the ancestors or lineal descent of that descendant can easily be traced using the unique parental ID for each generation working back to the oldest known generation ancestor.

Since additional research sources are continuously being discovered and made available. It is quite conceivable in the near future that a significant number of additional descendants may be uncovered. For that reason the author chose the above detailed method of generational identification and linking which would easily enable incorporating those additional descendants into the current identification scheme. This would facilitate publishing a supplement to the original book when sufficient new information warrants.

INTRODUCTION

It is important that the readers and users of this book be made aware of the ruling history and historical significance of the area where the subject Bruckman family originated from, as well as be provided some sense of the historical impact on this family as German Jewish people living in this constantly changing historical area which may have influenced their way of life and affected decisions made by some to bring about significant changes to improve their quality of life. Even though for some those changes forced them to abandon their homeland and ancestral family ties.

The two significant areas of origin for the subject Bruckman family have been identified as the present day towns of Loštice and Kroměříž located in the province of Morava in the Czech Republic. The Czech Republic government currently is in control of all of the historical records pertaining to these areas and is systematically making them available online through the efforts of the government archives. The following is a current map showing these two towns and their physical proximity to each other.

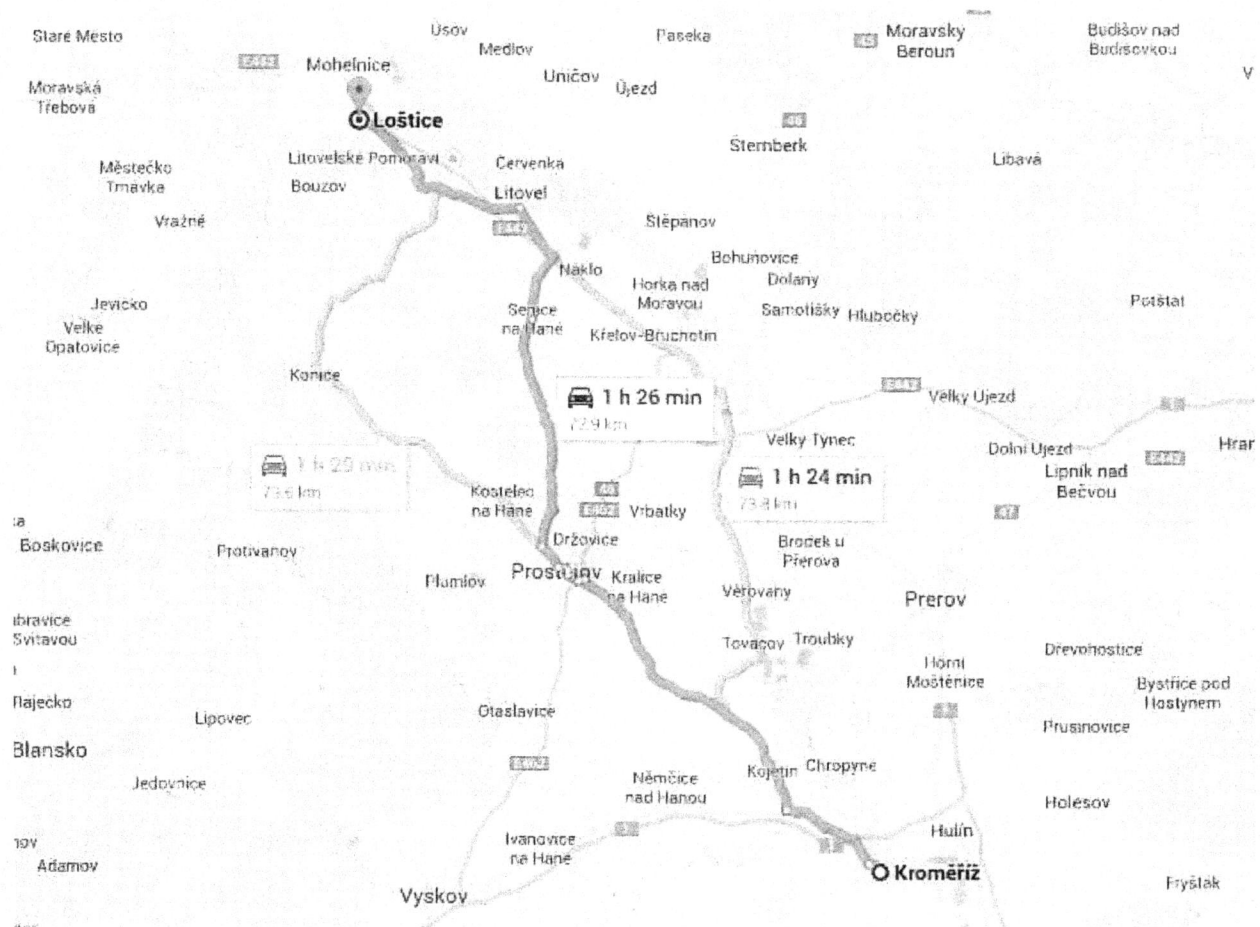

It is important to historical and genealogical research of these areas to know the English and German names for these locations as the earlier records tend to contain the German spellings and the record indexes may contain either the English or German spellings instead of the Czech spellings. The following is the three variations of spelling for comparison:

Language	Town Names	Province
Czech	Loštice and Kroměříž	Morava
German	Loschitz and Kremsier	Mähren
English	Lostice and Kromeriz	Moravia

It is equally important to understand that sometimes in records there is no reference to the province and instead reference will be made to the empire or kingdom to which it belonged. The Kingdom in this case is Bohemia (English), Böhmen (German) or Čechy (Czech) which is also the name of a province depending on the period of history. The Kingdom of Bohemia included both the provinces of Bohemia and Moravia, as well as other associated areas. So it must be understood that when these town names or people from them or the surrounding areas are referred to as Bohemian it is in reference to inclusion in or allegiance to the kingdom or empire and not the geographical province. This territory as part of the Kingdom of Bohemia was part of the Crown of Bohemia (1348–1918), part of the Holy Roman Empire (until 1806), part of the Habsburg Monarchy (1526–1804), Crown land of the Austrian Empire (1804–67) and part of Cisleithanian Austria-Hungary (1867–1918) .

Now that the areas of origin have been clearly identified it is necessary to provide their historical ruling evolution and its possible impact on the everyday lives of the subject family and its descendants.

The earliest Jewish records discovered so far place the family's earliest known beginnings within, or in the surrounding area of, the town of Kromeriz. At some point in time, generation 1 and at least one son migrated to the town of Lostice or its surrounding area, but before that, generation 1 is found to have married for the second time in Lostice in 1785.

The Jewish community of Kromeriz was among the oldest in Europe and its known general history until 1785 is as follows:

1322 the bishop of Olomouc (Olmuetz) was permitted to allow one Jew to settle in the town, exempt from servitude to the royal chamber (servi camerae regis). A community under the protection of the bishop grew up soon after; it remained under the protection of the successive bishops until 1848, and the synagogue and community house displayed the episcopal coat of arms, with a cross and cardinal's hat.

1340s A Jew sued a gentile before the town court.

1546 Jews moved to another part of the town because of conflicts with their neighbors.

1642 During the Thirty Years' War, the community was destroyed by the Swedes, an event mourned in several contemporary seli□ot.

1648 Kromeriz absorbed many refugees from the Chmielnicki massacres.

1670 Eight families were expelled from Vienna and settled in Kromeriz under the bishop's protection.

1676 Twenty-seven Jewish families lived in the town.

1689 Kromeriz was considered the most important and most affluent Moravian community after Mikulov (Nikolsburg) and from then until 1697 it was the seat of the country rabbinate.

1724 First census of all Jews in the Czech lands was carried out. Results of this census revealed approximately 30,000 Jews inhabited 168 towns and 672 villages in Bohemia and approximately 20,000 lived in Moravia, while 2,335 Jewish families (approximately 10,500 Jews) were registered in Prague.

1726 Habsburg ruler Charles VI, ordered that the number of Jewish families was limited by quota to 8,541 in Bohemia and 5,106 in Moravia. To enforce this quota (or "numerus clausus"), a so-called "Familianten" order was issued. According to this order, only the first-born son of each Jewish family was given permission to marry (called a "copulatio consensus"). The permits could also be sold if there were no son to inherit them. The Familianten order remained in force until 1848 and over time had caused many Jewish males to leave for places void of this unreasonable law.

1785 During the period of time in the 18th century leading up to this year the community of Kromeriz became very impoverished forcing many to leave in search of a more favorable and prosperous community. It is quite evident that the subject Bruckman family was among those who migrated to Lostice as a result of the aforementioned reasons.

The Jewish community of Lostice was also among the oldest in Europe and its known general history until the mid 19th century is as follows:

1781-88 Reforms declared by the Emperor Joseph II began to remove the most discriminatory laws, made education accessible for all and prepared the conditions for integration of Jews into society.

1782 A Jewish school opened in Lostice and by request of the Jewish community, a local Christian schoolteacher, Josef Cap, began to teach there.

1787 Emperor Joseph II, ruler of the Austro-Hungarian Empire, who controlled a substantial part of Europe at the time, issued a decree that required all Jews to register a permanent family surname, and they required that this surname be German. This was the first country in Europe to create such a law.

1793 A fire, which started in the Jewish quarter, spread to the town and destroyed 38 houses.

1805-06 A synagogue built of masonry in the Classicist style replaced a former wooden structure and is preserved to the present day. This synagogue was used by the Nazis as a warehouse during WW II. It became a municipal museum in 1958 and is owned by the city today. It is used now as a cultural and educational center run by Respect and Tolerance, a foundation dedicated to documenting, researching and teaching about Jewish history and culture in northern Moravia, which oversaw the renovation. After ten years of work, restoration of the synagogue in the town of Loštice has been completed, a milestone that was celebrated with a gala event on October 5, 2014 (The main restoration was completed in 2011). The following photo is the synagogue in Loštice as it appeared on 06 Oct. 2014. The photo was taken by William "Bill" Richard Griffith, a Bruckman descendant, and his wife Julie while visiting Loštice during the 10th anniversary celebration of the restoration of the synagogue.

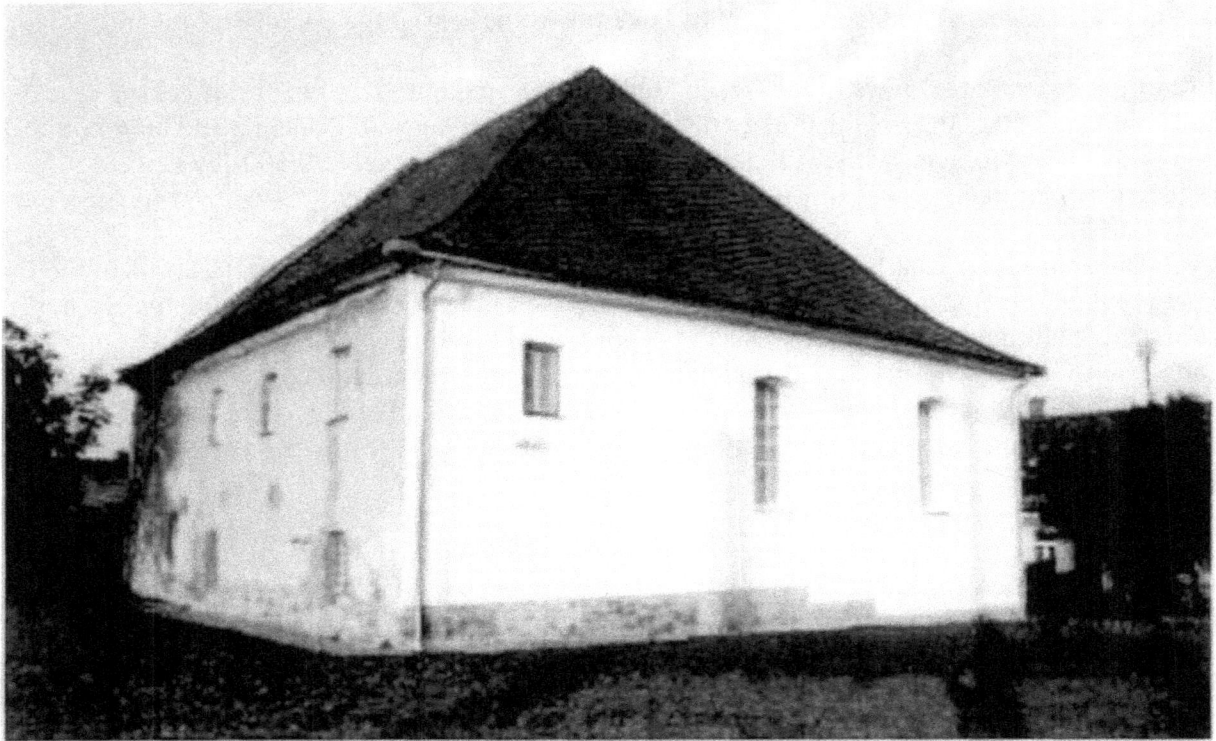

1808 All old taxation duties were discharged, while three others were re-established as a family tax, property tax and food tax. The corporation, "K.K. Direktion des Judischen Steuerfalls", was in charge of collecting these taxes

1836 The Official Seal of The Jewish Community of Lostice was created and required to be used on all Jewish documents by the state administration.

1848-49 Revolutionary events caused a major reorganization of the state administration and an improvement of rights for all citizens.

1867 Jews attained civil rights with a final amendment allowing Jews to relocate freely, choose any profession and marry without restrictions. Feudal ownership was dismantled and Lostice became a free town. Christian and Jewish communities created a joint municipal administration. There were 483 Jews in Lostice, which represented about 17 % of the inhabitants.

Raymond Clyde Lantz

References: 57- Moravia, 57-Bohemia, 57-Kroměříž, 57-Loštice, 57-Czech Republic, 57-Austrian Empire, 60, 61, 62, 63, 64, 65

PROLOGUE

Tracing Jacob George Bruckman's history and ancestry has been a challenging and elusive task. The information available from 19th century Pennsylvania census records listed him as having been born in Austria or Bohemia and indicated that he was a medical doctor. There was a clue that he had a Jewish background: his granddaughter, Fannie Bruckman Griffith (who was born several years after Jacob died), spoke in her later years of having visited her Jewish cousins in New York when she was a child.

The search for Jacob turned up another Bruckman—Philip, a well-documented Jew who lived in New York from 1842 until his death in 1874. Philip was an early member of the oldest Jewish service organization, B'nai B'rith (Sons of the Covenant), and his wife, Hennretta, was the founder of a Jewish women's organization, The Independent Order of True Sisters. Philip had emigrated from Bohemia in the same year as Jacob, and was also a medical doctor. Born in December of 1797, Philip was a little more than two years older than Jacob; could they have been brothers?

The answer to that question was hard to come by. Two of Jacob's descendants, Ray Lantz and Bill Griffith were independently working on the problem and both had hired genealogists in Europe to look for Jacob, particularly searching for his ancestors and also where he had trained to become a medical doctor.

Going on a hunch that Jacob was Philip's brother, Bill asked his genealogist in Prague to check on records in Pilsen. Pilsen was a town listed as the departure point in Bohemia for Philipp and Henreitta Bruckman when they immigrated to the US. The researcher, David Kohout, found birth records for Alexander Bruckman the son of Philip and Henreitta who was born in Pilsen. The birth record for Alexander recorded that the father of Philip Bruckman was Moshe Bruckman who lived in Lostice. Bill turned this information over to Ray who asked his people to locate this town of Lostice. They determined Lostice to be located in Moravia. They also found records from Lostice indicating that Moshe had a son Philipp, born in 1797, and a son Jacob, born in 1800, so the link was made. Subsequently Ray located another cousin who had in his position the medical license of Jacob Bruckman and it states that he was from Lostice so we had added proof that we had located the right Jacob Bruckman.

A birth record for Philip's son, Alexander, was located and it included the information that Philip was a medical doctor and was the son of "Moise Brukman" whose occupation was listed as "Schulsinger" (Synagogue Cantor) in Loštice. Jacob's birth record had been located and it listed his father as Moise, the Schulsinger in Loštice. Thus, Philip and Jacob were, indeed, brothers.

Knowing that Jacob was the son of Moise, it was possible to trace back one more generation to Moishe's father, Lazarus Brŭckmann who was born in either 1722 or 1727 in Kremsier (now Kromeriź, Czech Republic), a town located about 80 miles southeast of Loštice. The information gleaned about Lazarus was found in registers of his second marriage and his death, so currently nothing is known about his first wife who would have been the mother of Moishe and his brother Jacob.

Peggy Griffith Covert

CHAPTER 1

I LAZARUS BRÜCKMANN

LAZARUS BRÜCKMANN was born 1722/7 Kremsier, Böhmen, Austria (now Kromeríž, Czech Republic) and died 14 Apr 1795 in House #10, Loschitz, Böhmen, Austria (now Loštice, Czech Republic) of old age. He married (1) _____ before 1764. He married (2) SARA SABL on 03 Nov 1785 in House #10, Loschitz, Böhmen, Austria (now Loštice, Czech Republic). She was born in 1740 and died on 11 Mar 1799 in Loschitz, Böhmen, Austria of tuberculosis. He is called a "beglaubter" when appearing in the synagogue records. This has been determined to mean as the author understands is someone that you can believe or one that believes. Also the notaries in Germany and Austria are commonly called Beglaubters. This family was Jewish German and lived in House #10 as indicated in all of the vital record entries shown below recorded in the synagogue record books. The House # found in these records is new to the author and in many cases is a significant help to the researcher. The researcher must also beware the normally several families often reside in each house or dwelling. The birth place of LAZARUS BRÜCKMANN is based on his 2nd marriage and death entries recorded at Loštice. In which he is recorded as from Kremsier which is about 80 miles southeast of Loschitz. Historic records for Kremsier attest that in the period most of the 18th century prior to 1785 the community of Kremsier became very impoverished forcing many to leave in search of more favorable and prosperous community. It is quite evident that the subject Bruckman family was among those who migrated to Lostice for this reason. However, so far no evidence has been found to ascertain the exact year that members of this family settled in Lostice, but certainly prior to 1785 when the aforementioned marriage occurred.

The Loštice synagogue record books begin 1765 for births, 1784 for marriages and 1784 for deaths. Many of the earlier events, as late as 1790, were entered in the books retroactively and many of those events occurring of that period were also forgotten and never entered. In 1544 Benes, a man of Jewish faith, bought a house in the town and is the oldest record of a Jewish settlement in Lostice. At this time Lostice was a part of the Bouzov estate and its feudal owner was Vaclav Haugvic of Biskupice. A decade later in 1554 a Jewish cemetery was established by the road to Palonin. Not long after about 1560 the first wooden synagogue was built in the Jewish quarter near the parish church.

Children of LAZARUS BRÜCKMANN and (?) are:

i. MOISHE BRÜCKMANN (II) See Following.

ii. JACOB BRÜCKMANN (III) was born probably in Kremsier, Böhmen, Austria. Currently there are no known descendants.

Ref: 22, 60, 61, 62, 63, 64, 65, 66, 67, 68

LAZARUS BRÜCKMANN and SARA SABL marriage record

LAZARUS BRÜCKMANN death record

SARA (SABL) BRÜCKMANN death record

2

MOISHE BRÜCKMANN was born probably in 1764 Kremsier, Böhmen, Austria and died 13 May 1800 in Loschitz, Böhmen, Austria of tuberculosis, House # not given, assumed to be #10. He married RACHEL LÖBL on 22 May 1790 in House #10, Loschitz, Böhmen, Austria, daughter of ARON LÖBL and SAREL _____. She was born on 15 Feb 1772 in House #10, Loschitz, Böhmen, Austria and died on Feb 1804 in House #12, Loschitz, Böhmen, Austria of tuberculosis. Like his father, MOISHE BRÜCKMANN is found in the synagogue records as a "beglaubter" understood by the author to mean someone that you can believe or one that believes. He is listed as deceased and a *Schulsinger* or Cantor in Loschitz, Böhmen, Austria in the birth record of his grandson ALEXANDER BRUCKMAN, son of DR. PHILIP/PINCUS BRUCKMAN.

The author believes that their two sons DR. PHILIP BRUCKMAN and DR. JACOB GEORGE BRUCKMAN eventually fled from their homeland in Böhmen, Austria to escape the continuous and rising levels of anti-Semitism throughout their native country and neighboring countries. They chose emigration to America where it was known to be a more Jewish friendly and tolerant place.

(Hebrew Name Origin/Meaning: Moshe was the greatest prophet ever, who led the Jewish people in the Exodus from Egypt, and at the receiving of the Torah at Mount Sinai. Moshe means "drawn out [of the water]" (Exodus 2:10), for in a deeper sense, Moshe's destiny was to draw the Jewish people out of slavery. (variations: Moishe, Moses))

Children of MOISHE BRÜCKMANN and RACHEL LÖBL are:

  i. LÖBL BRÜCKMANN (A) See Chapter 2 for descendants.

  ii. JUDITH BRÜCKMANN (B) See Chapter 3 for descendants.

  iii. LAZARUS BRÜCKMANN (C) See Chapter 4 for descendants.

  iv. PHILIP/PINCUS BRUCKMAN (D) See Chapter 5 for descendants.

  v. JACOB GEORGE BRUCKMAN (E) See Chapter 6 for descendants.

Ref: 4-17th Ward New York City New York Co NY, 15-1855 New York City New York Co NY, 17, 18, 19, 20, 22, 67, 68

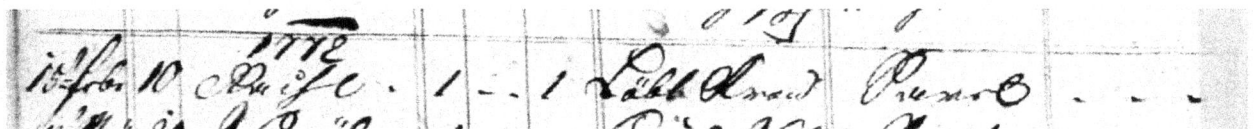

RACHEL LÖBL birth record

MOISHE BRÜCKMANN and RACHEL LÖBL marriage record

MOISHE BRÜCKMANN death record

RACHEL LÖBL death record

CHAPTER 2

A LÖBL BRÜCKMANN II

LÖBL BRÜCKMANN was born on 15 Mar 1792 in House #10, Loschitz, Böhmen, Austria (now Loštice, Czech Republic). He married KATY COHN on 22 ??? 1822 in Loschitz, Böhmen, Austria (now Loštice, Czech Republic), daughter of ? and ?. She was born 1800 in Loschitz, Böhmen, Austria (now Loštice, Czech Republic).

Children of LÖBL BRÜCKMANN and KATY COHN had the following children:

i. RACHEL BRÜCKMANN (A1) was born on 04 Feb 1824 in House (?), Loschitz, Böhmen, Austria (now Loštice, Czech Republic).

ii. DAUGHTER BRÜCKMANN (A2) was born and died on 05 Apr 1840 in House #9, Loschitz, Böhmen, Austria (now Loštice, Czech Republic), stillborn.

Ref: 22

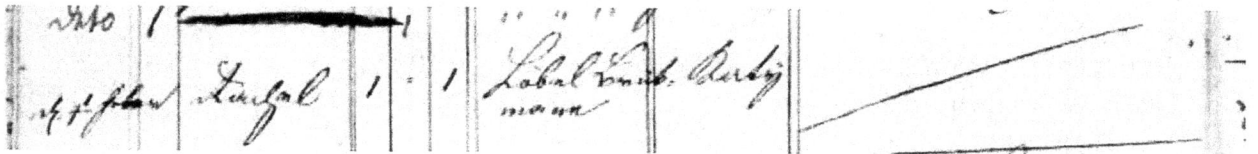

RACHEL BRÜCKMANN birth record

DAUGHTER BRÜCKMANN stillborn birth record

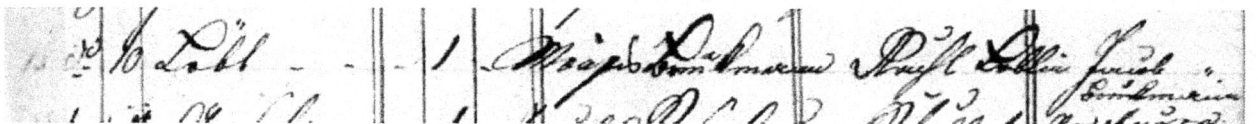

LÖBL BRÜCKMANN birth record

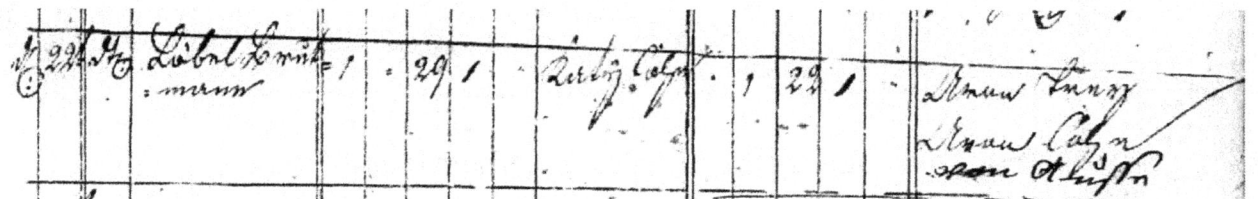

LÖBL BRÜCKMANN and KATY COHN marriage record

CHAPTER 3

B JUDITH BRÜCKMANN II

JUDITH BRÜCKMANN was born on 15 Mar 1794 in House #10, Loschitz, Böhmen, Austria (now Loštice, Czech Republic) and died on 28 May 1874 in Jewish Cemetery, Loschitz, Böhmen, Austria (now Loštice, Czech Republic). She was buried in Jewish Cemetery in Loschitz, Böhmen, Austria (now Loštice, Czech Republic). All of her children are listed as illegitimate in the birth records and a father's name is not listed. Given to Jewish custom or law if a Jewish woman's husband is not Jewish then the child is said not to have a father and therefore the father's name would not be recorded in the birth record.

Children of JUDITH BRÜCKMANN and _____ are:

i. MOJSES BRÜCKMANN (B1) was born on 02 Sep 1818 in House (?), Loschitz, Böhmen, Austria (now Loštice, Czech Republic).

ii. SOLOMON BRÜCKMANN (B2) was born on 02 Aug 1820 in House (?), Loschitz, Böhmen, Austria (now Loštice, Czech Republic).

iii. JUDITH RACHEL BRÜCKMANN (B3) was born on 10 May 1824 in House (?), Loschitz, Böhmen, Austria (now Loštice, Czech Republic).

iv. RACHEL BRÜCKMANN (B4)

v. SAMUEL BRÜCKMANN (B5) was born on 28 May 1826 in House (?), Loschitz, Böhmen, Austria (now Loštice, Czech Republic) and died on 22 Mar 1873 in House (?), Loschitz, Böhmen, Austria (now Loštice, Czech Republic). He was buried in Jewish Cemetery in Loschitz, Böhmen, Austria (now Loštice, Czech Republic).

Ref: 22

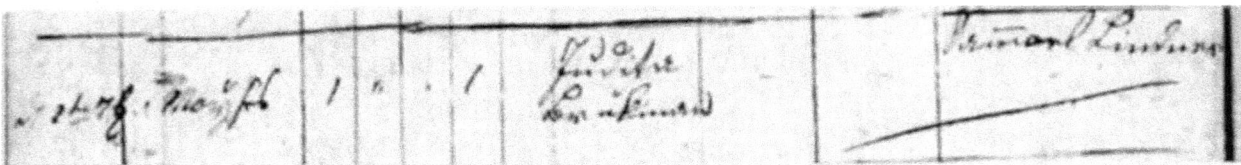

MOJSES BRÜCKMANN birth record

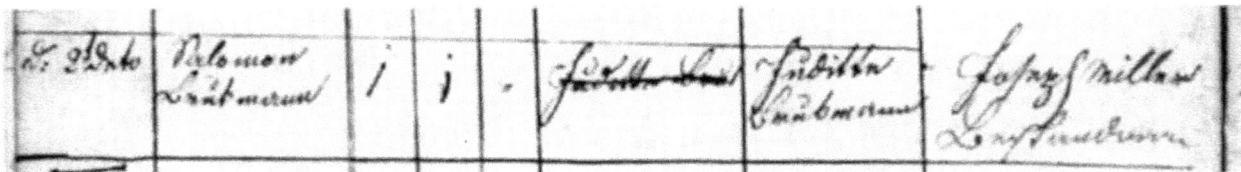

SOLOMON BRÜCKMANN birth record

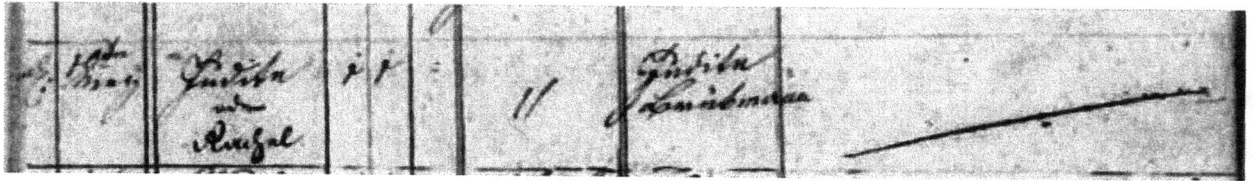

JUDITH RACHEL BRÜCKMANN birth record

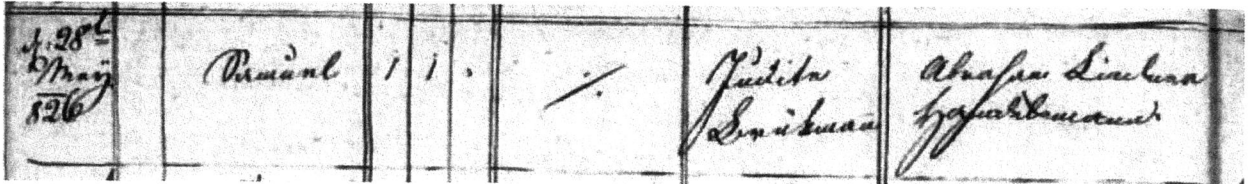

SAMUEL BRÜCKMANN birth record

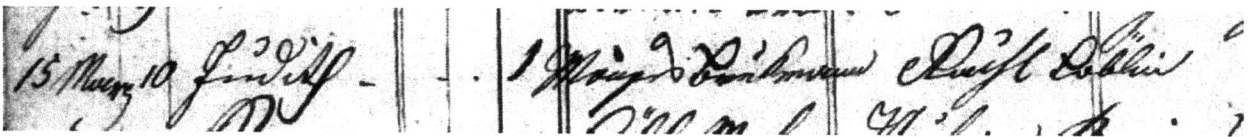

JUDITH BRÜCKMANN (mother) birth record

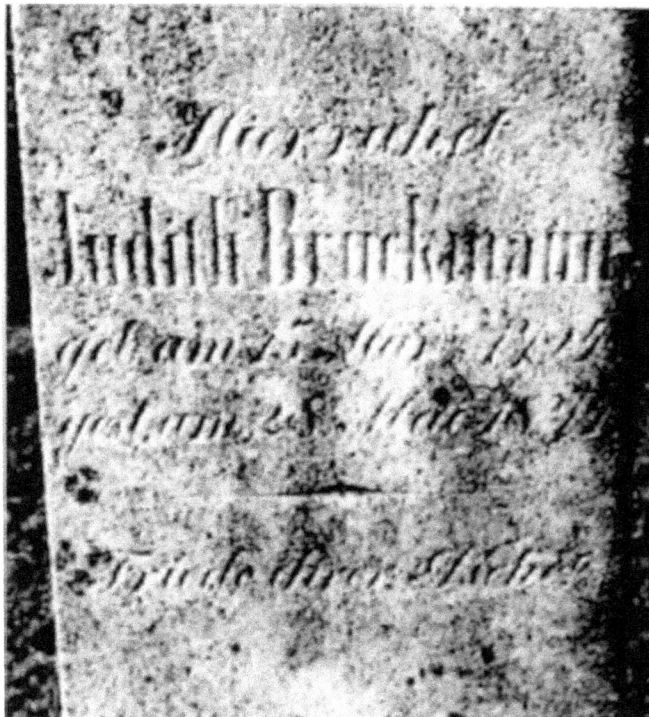

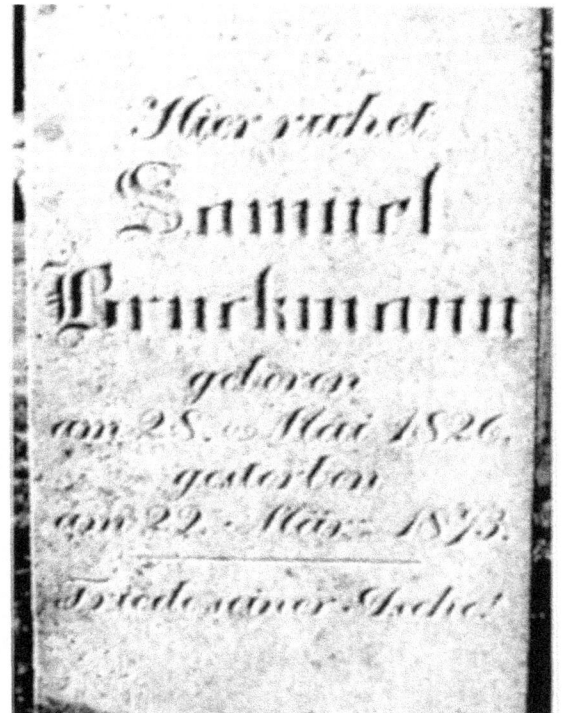

Gravestones above are that of Judith Bruckmann and her son Samuel Bruckmann located in the Jewish cemetery at Loštice, Czech Republic. The inscriptions written in Hebrew are located on the opposite faces of the gravestones. (Photos by William "Bill" Richard Griffith)

MORITZ BRÜCKMANN death Loschitz death index book

B42 FANNY BRÜCKMANN B4

FANNY BRÜCKMANN was born on 20 May 1846 in House #17, Loschitz, Böhmen, Austria (now Loštice, Czech Republic). She married ISRAEL KOHN in House #?, Loschitz, Böhmen, Austria (now Loštice, Czech Republic). After the death of her husband she was approved to change her surname back to her maiden name in a decree of 23 Feb 1912 in Brünn (Brno).

Ref: 22

FANNY BRÜCKMANN birth record

CHAPTER 4

C LAZARUS BRÜCKMANN II

LAZARUS BRÜCKMANN was born on 01 Feb 1796 in House #10, Loschitz, Böhmen, Austria (now Loštice, Czech Republic). Currently there are no known descendants.

Ref: 22

CHAPTER 5

D PHILIP/PINCUS BRUCKMAN II

DR. PHILIP/PINCUS BRUCKMAN was born on 26 Dec 1797 in House #6, Loschitz, Böhmen, Austria (now Loštice, Czech Republic) and died 07 Nov 1874 in Manhattan, New York, NY. He married HENNRETTA KAHN about 1831 in Böhmen, Austria (now Czech Republic), daughter of SIMON KAHN and AMALIE DATTELGEWEIG. She was born in Apr 1810 in Pilsen, Böhmen, Austria (now Plzeň, Czech Republic) and died 07 Apr 1888 in Manhattan, New York, NY. They came from Austria via Bremen, Germany aboard the ship *Elard* and arrived at New York City, NY on 27 Aug 1842. He was naturalized on 22 Oct 1847 in New York City, NY. They resided at 184 Essex Street, New York City, NY in 1848-1849 and were enumerated in the federal census in 1850 in 17th Ward, New York City, New York Co., NY and in the state census in 1855 in New York City, New York Co., NY. His occupation upon arrival was listed as physician, but in 1855 he is listed as conducting a jewelry business.

Before coming to America DR. PHILIP/PINCUS BRUCKMAN was a practicing physician in Pilsen, Böhmen, Austria, where his family also resided. It is yet uncertain where he attended medical school or when he began his practice in Pilsen.

After arrival in America the family was quickly accepted as members of New York City's German Jewish elite. They began immediately to support the charitable efforts on behalf of their less well-off fellow immigrants, and participating in the community's cultural life. These efforts facilitated DR. PHILIP BRUCKMAN becoming part of a group of German immigrants that founded the Mendelssohnian Society, a religious confraternity with reform goals and later known as Temple Emanu-El (God is with us). This new association eventually became the inspiration for the establishment of the B'nai B'rith (Children of the Covenant), a secular Jewish fraternal order, in 1843, the oldest Jewish service organization in the world. As mentioned this family's charitable efforts were a family effort and it is only expected that HENRIETTA BRUCKMAN would have wished to be by her husband's side in the pursuit of those efforts. However, share interest fell on deaf ears as the B'nai B'rith continued to refuse to accept female members. She not being one to be easily prevented from achieving her goals in support of a worthwhile cause, she would usually find a way to succeed when she put her mind to it. In 1846, Henrietta Bruckman, mustering support from among her friends, proposed the creation of a female counterpart to the B'nai B'rith open exclusively to women. This effort was openly supported by her husband. His support aided her in also to seek and gain the support of his business partner Dr. James Mitchel, Rabbi Dr. Leo *Merzbacher , the minister of Emanu-El, and a number of influential members of the B'nai B'rith and Temple Emanu-El. At the first meeting of the Emanuel Lodge of the Unabhängiger Orden Treuer Schwestern (Independent Order of True Sisters) she was installed as its first president. Under her leadership the order quickly became a Model of Modernity for Nineteenth Century American Jewish Womanhood. Through her efforts her installation as president of the Order established the first fraternal organization in America open exclusively to women.

WILLIAM "BILL" RICHARD GRIFFITH, a descendant, had reported to the author that: "My grandmother FANNIE BRUCKMAN told me that as a child she would travel to New York and visit her Jewish cousins. I asked her who these people were and she didn't know. Her father FRANKLIN DAVID BRUCKMAN died when she was 10 or 11 and the visits stopped." The Jewish component connection is further strengthened through DNA testing. The author's test results reveal an estimated 11% ethnic makeup of Jewish Ashkenazi Diaspora and the author's cousin WILLIAM RICHARD GRIFFITH results indicate an estimated 4-5% ethnic makeup of Jewish Ashkenazi Diaspora also. In short this significant new information led to the discovery of DR. PHILIP BRUCKMAN as the brother of DR. JACOB GEORGE BRUCKMAN (E) (see Chapter 6), and subsequent significant discovery of the birth record of DR. PHILIP BRUCKMAN's son ALEXANDER BRUCKMAN (D5) (see following), that names the parents of DR. PHILIP BRUCKMAN and HENNRETTA KAHN, and more. The birth record has led to the discovery of the birth records and ancestors of DR. PHILIP BRUCKMAN and his siblings, including his brother DR. JACOB GEORGE BRUCKMAN (E) (see Chapter 6) great grandfather of the cousin and the author's 2nd great grandfather.

Children of PHILIP BRUCKMAN and HENNRETTA KAHN are:

 i. THERESA BRUCKMAN (D1)

 ii. HERMAN BRUCKMAN (D2)

 iii. ALOYS "LOUIS" BRUCKMAN (D3)

 iv. SIGMOND "SIMON" BRUCKMAN (D4) was born in 1837 in Böhmen, Austria (now Czech Republic).

 v. ALEXANDER BRUCKMAN (D5)

 vi. EMILY BRUCKMAN (D6) was born in 1843 in New York City, New York Co., NY.

 vii. JAMES BRUCKMAN (D7)

 viii. JOHN BRUCKMAN (D8)

 ix. FREDERICK BRUCKMAN (D9)

 x. CHARLES BRUCKMAN (DA)

Ref: 22, 17, 18, 19, 20, 4-17th Ward NYC NY Co NY F1294, 5-1st Dist 16th Ward NYC NY Co NY F1817, 6-16th Dist 19th Ward NY Co NY F173, 7-San Francisco San Francisco Co CA F199, 15-1855 8th Dist 17th Ward NYC NY Co, 32-ED 8 Ward 16 NYC NY Co, 69, 70, 57-B'nai B'rith, 71, 72, 73, 27-D-HB-11099, 27-D-PB-191001

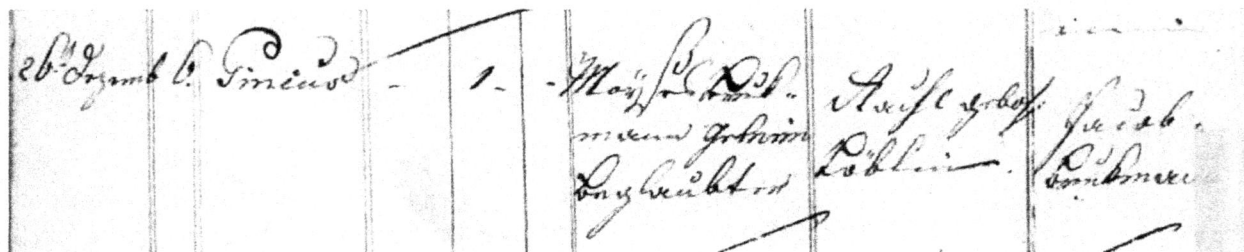

PHILIP BRÜCKMANN birth record

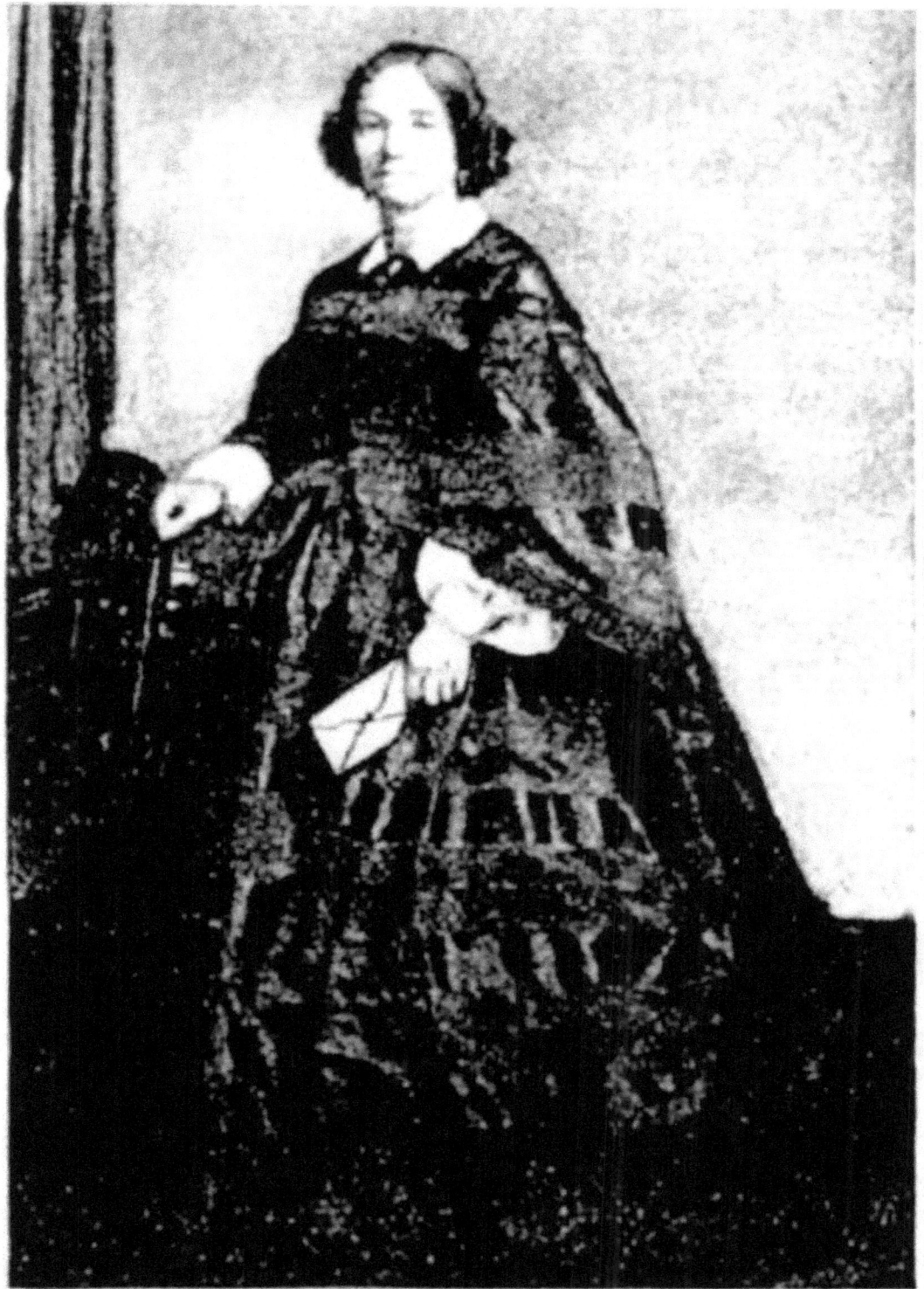

Henriette Bruckmann, founder of the Independent Order of True Sisters. Courtesy of Archives of Congregation Emanu-El, New York, New York.

At a Surrogate's Court held in and for
the County of New York at the Surrogate's
Office in the City of New York, on the
Eleventh day of June in the year 1888.

Present,

Hon. Rastus S. Ransom,
Surrogate.

In the Matter of Proving the
Last Will and Testament
of
Henriette Brückmann
Deceased.

The Citation herein having been duly issued, served
waived and returned, & Van Wyck Esq. appearing
for the Petitioner, and the Surrogate having on his
own motion appointed John H. Rogan Esq. Special
Guardian of the infants herein and the allegations
of the said parties appearing having been heard,
and the proofs having been duly taken by the
Surrogate, among other things as to the execution
of said instrument, bearing date Sept. 12th 1876
and the Probate of the said Will not having
been contested, and it appearing to the Surrogate
that the Will was duly executed, and that the
Testatrix at the time of executing it was in all
respects competent to make a Will and not under
restraint: it is Ordered, Adjudged and Decreed,
that the instrument offered for probate herein be
and the same hereby is admitted to probate as
the Last Will and Testament of the said deceased
valid to pass real and personal property, and
that Letters Testamentary be issued thereon to
the executors who may qualify thereunder.
And that said John H. Rogan the special
Guardian appointed for the infants herein be and

15

he did so at the request of said decedent, and in her presence.

Louis Heilprin.

Witness affirmed and examined }
before me this 9th day of June 1888 }
Charles H. Beckett
Assistant to the Surrogate
New York County.

City, County and State of New York, SS:
Solomon B. Livingston
of New York City, being duly affirmed as a witness in the above entitled matter, and examined on behalf of the applicant to prove said will, says: I was well acquainted with Henriette Bruckmann now deceased.

I knew the above named decedent for more than twenty years before her death. The subscription of the name of said decedent to the instrument now shown to me and offered for probate as her last will and testament, and bearing date the twelfth day of September in the year one thousand eight hundred and seventy six, was made by the decedent at the City of New York, on the twelfth day of September in the year one thousand eight hundred and seventy six in the presence of myself and Louis Heilprin the other subscribing witness.

At the time of such subscription the said decedent declared the said instrument so subscribed by her to be her last will and testament: and I thereupon signed my name as a witness at the end of said instrument, at the request of said decedent, and in her presence.

The said decedent, at the time of so executing said instrument, was upwards of the age of twenty one years, and of sound mind, memory and understanding, and not under any restraint, or in any respect incompetent to make a will. I also saw said Louis Heilprin the other attesting witness sign his name as a witness at the end of said will and knew that he did so at the request of said decedent, and in her presence.

S B Livingston.

Witness Affirmed and Examined
before me, this 9t day of June 1888
Charles H Beckett
Assistant to the Surrogate
New York County.

I, Henriette Bruckmann, widow of Dr Philet
Bruckmann deceased, of the City of New
York, do make, ordain, publish and declare
this to be my last will and testament hereby
revoking and annulling all former wills by
me made
First. After the payment of my just debts I
order and direct my executors hereinafter
named or such of them as may qualify, to
divide the residue of the estate of which I
may die seised, or in any way possessed,
into ten equal shares as near as may be,
and to dispose of the same as follows to wit
Second. I give and bequeath one equal share
to each of my children living at my death
and to the representatives of such of them as
shall have died, except that in case my
daughter Emily, should die before me, her
share shall not be given to her children, but
shall be divided equally among the remaining
children and their representatives entitled
to take under the provisions of this will; and
further it is my will that the share of the
children of my son Louis, deceased, be
given to his widow Theresa Bruckmann
reposing full confidence, in her, that she
will keep or dispose of the same for the
benefit of said children in accordance with
my wish.
Third. In case of the death of any of my children
leaving no issue or representatives it is my
will that the share or shares of such child
or children be divided equally among the
remaining children and their representatives
entitled to take under the provisions of this
my will.
Fourth. Should any of my children decline
to take the share which falls to them,
under this will, the same shall be given
in the discretion of my executors to such

other of my children who shall be in needy circum-
stances or in want of same or be divided up
among the remaining persons entitled to take
under the provisions of this will, and in
manner herein provided.

Fifth. I nominate and appoint my two youngest
sons Charles and Frederick, Executors to
carry out the provision of this my will.

In Witness Whereof I have hereunto set my hand
and seal this twelfth day of September 1876.

Henriette Bruckmann (LS).

Signed, Sealed, Published and declared by the
testatrix as and for her last will and testament
in our presence who at her request in her presence
and in the presence of each other have affixed
our names hereto as subscribing witnesses

Louis Heilprin Residence 24 Beekman Pl. New York City.
S. B. Livingston Residence 214 East 53d St. NY City

D1 THERESA BRUCKMAN D

THERESA BRUCKMAN was born in 1832 in Böhmen, Austria (now Czech Republic). She married MORRIS FALLENBURGH in NYC, NY Co., NY. He was born 1832 in Austria.

Children of THERESA BRUCKMAN and MORRIS FALLENBURGH are:

i. WILLIAM FALLENBURGH (D11) was born in 1852 in NYC, NY Co., NY.

ii. LOUISA FALLENBURGH (D12) was born in 1854 in NYC, NY Co., NY.

Ref: 32-ED 8 Ward 16 NYC NY Co

D2 HERMAN BRUCKMAN D

HERMAN BRUCKMAN was born in 1834 in Böhmen, Austria (now Czech Republic). He married DELFINA L. MALDONADO on 8 Sep 1866 in Storey Co., NV. She was born 1842 in Mexico.

Children of HERMANN BRUCKMAN and are:

i. ALBERT BRUCKMAN (D21) was born in 1860 in NV.

ii. EDWARD BRUCKMAN (D22) was born in 1861 in NV.

iii. THERESA BRUCKMAN (D23) was born in 1867 in CA.

Ref: 6-Ward 2 San Francisco San Francisco Co CA F1570, 28-09 Sep1866

D3 ALOYS "LOUIS" BRUCKMAN D

ALOYS "LOUIS" BRUCKMAN was born on 21 May 1835 in Böhmen, Austria (now Czech Republic) and died before 12 Sep 1876. He married THERESA EIDLITZ in NYC, NY Co., NY, daughter of ABRAHAM "ADOLF" EIDLITZ and JUDITH (JULIA) LOBISCH. She was born in Oct 1836 in Austria and died 19 Mar 1908 in Manhattan, NY.

Children of LOUIS BRUCKMAN and THERESA EIDLITZ are:

i. MATILDA H. BRUCKMAN (D31) was born in Jul 1861 in NYC, NY Co., NY and died 07 Sep 1911 in NYC, NY Co., NY. She was never married.

ii. ARTHUR BRUCKMAN (D32) was born on 20 Jul 1863 in NYC, NY Co., NY. He married (1) MARTHA COHEN on 05 May 1892 in Manhattan, NYC, NY Co., NY, daughter of MOSES S. COHEN and DONA BENRIMO. She was born in 1863 in NYC, NY Co., NY. He married (2) JENNIE LEVY on 05 Jan 1905 in Manhattan, NYC, NY Co., NY, daughter of ISAAC LEVY and RACHEL PINNER. She was born in 1863 in NYC, NY Co., NY.

iii. CAROLINE BRUCKMAN (D33) was born in Oct 1865 in NYC, NY Co., NY. She was never married.

iv. LUDMILLA BRUCKMAN (D34) was born in Nov 1868 in NYC, NY Co., NY. She was never married.

v. LOUISA ALICE BRUCKMAN (D35) was born in 16 Mar 1872 in Manhattan, NYC, NY Co., NY. She was never married.

Ref: 39, 6-NYC NY Co NY F325, 7-NYC NY Co NY F266, 8-NYC NY Co NY F115, 38, 37, 40, 15-1915-NYC NY NY H170, 75-Manhatten NY NY Pg 26

24185 – Aug. 14. 1872   H. Anslice & Co., Stationers, 23 Nassau Street, N. Y.

United States of America,

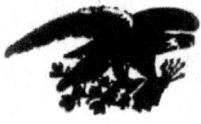

State of New-York, ss.

By this Public Instrument be it known to all whom

the same doth or may in any wise concern, that I, *Alexander Robertson Rodgers* Public Notary
in and for the State of **NEW-YORK**, by Letters Patent under the Great Seal of the said
State, duly commissioned and sworn, **Do Hereby Certify**, That the persons named in the
annexed papers, appeared before me, and being duly sworn according to law, each subscribed
the declaration made by him respectively, which I deem sufficient proof of the citizenship
of *Louis Bruckman* who subscribed the annexed
affidavit. And I Certify the annexed description of his person to be correct.

        In Testimony whereof, I have subscribed my name, and
caused my Notarial Seal of Office to be hereunto affixed
the *thirteenth* day of *August*
in the year of our Lord one thousand eight hundred and
seventy *two* and of Independence the

                  AR Rodgers
                  NOTARY PUBLIC.

STATE OF NEW-YORK,
City & County of New York ss.

     I, *Louis Bruckman* do swear that I was born in
Bohemia in the Empire of Austria
on or about the **21st** day of **May** — **1835** that I am a
naturalized and loyal citizen of the United States, and am about to travel abroad,
with my wife and five minor children and that I am
   Sworn to before me, this 13 day   the identical person described
of *August*   1872   in the certificate of naturalization
       AR Rodgers   herewith presented.
        Notary Public.   *L Bruckman*

STATE OF NEW-YORK,
City & County of New York ss.

     I, *Henry Lane* — do swear that I am acquainted
with the above named *Louis Bruckman* — and with the facts above
stated by him, and that the same are true to the best of my knowledge and belief

     Sworn to before me, this 13th day
of *August* — 1872   *Henry H. Lane*
       AR Rodgers
        Notary Public.

Description of *Louis Bruckman*

Age	37 years.	Mouth	medium
Stature	5 feet 8½ inches, English.	Chin	round
Forehead	high	Hair	Brown
Eyes	gray	Complexion	florid
Nose	prominent	Face	oval

                  AR Rodgers
                  Notary Public

D5 ALEXANDER BRUCKMAN D

ALEXANDER BRUCKMAN was born on 10 Nov 1840 in Pilsen, Böhmen, Austria (now Plzeň, Czech Republic). He married (1) LILLIE E. SMITH on 25 Jun 1867 in Victoria, British Columbia, Canada, daughter of GEORGE SMITH and HELEN _____. She was born in NY. He married (2) ESTHER MCCARN. She was born in May 1850 in NY.

Child of ALEXANDER BRUCKMAN and ESTHER MCCARN is:

i. GRACE HERMANITA BRUCKMAN (D51)

Ref: 8-Ward 4 Ogden Weber Co UT F336, 9-Palo Alto, Santa Clara Co CA F260, 10-Palo Alto, Santa Clara Co CA F516, 41, 73

ALEXANDER BRUCKMAN birth record
Registers of Jewish Religious Communities in the Czech regions
The Czech National Archives
(1735) 1784 - 1949 (1960)

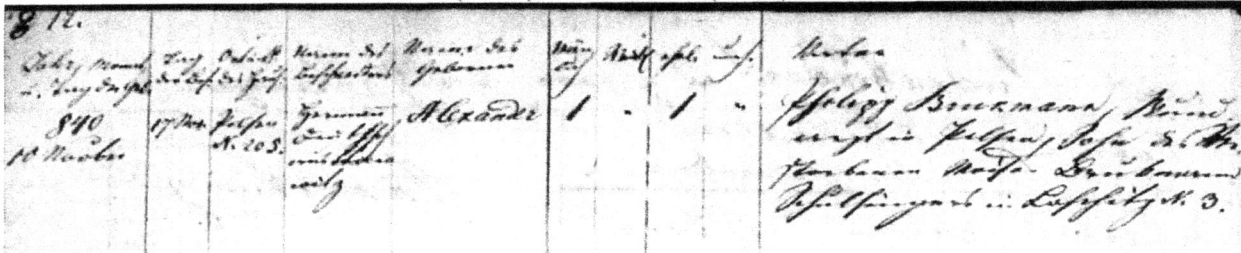

Translation:　　The date of the birth: on 10th November 1840
The date of circumsise: on 17th November
The birthplace: Pilsen House #205
The circumcise done by: Hermann Deutsch from....... *(? – illegible)*
The name: **Alexander**, male, born in lawful wedlock
The father: Philipp **Brukman**, „wundartz = *medical doctor* in Pilsen, the son of deceased Moise Brukman, „Schulsinger = *Cantor* in Lohchitz = *Loštice* # 3

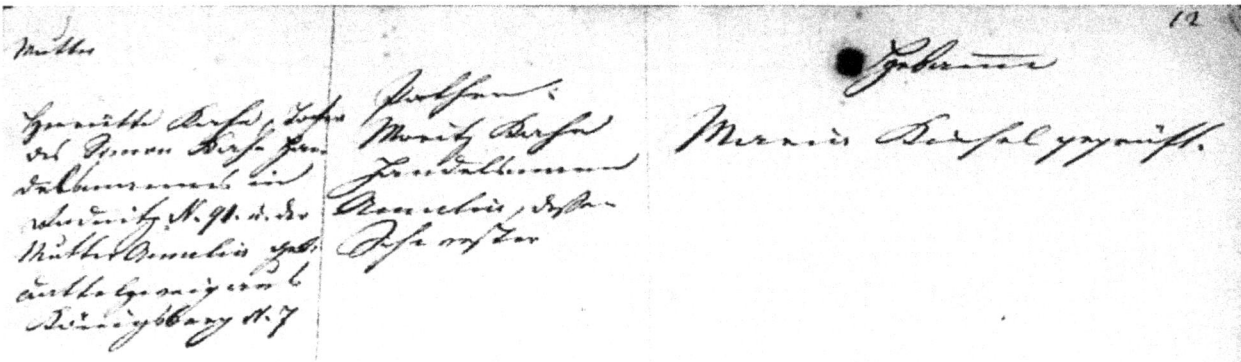

Translation:　　The mother: Henriette Kahn, the daughter of Simon Kahn, the merchant in Radnitz House #91 *(or #90?)* and of the mother Amalie nee Dattelgeweig? From Königsberg House #7

The godparents: Moritz Kahn, the merchant Amalie, his wife
The midwife: Marie Kasel (?), tested ."

D7 JAMES BRUCKMAN D

JAMES BRUCKMAN was born in 1845 in New York City, New York Co., NY. He married CLARA NETTIE HILL on 13 Apr 1887 in Denver, Arapahoe Co., CO. She was born on 15 Dec 1858 in IA and died 31 Dec 1950 in Los Angeles Co., CA. She is buried in Forest Lawn Memorial Park, Glendale, Los Angeles Co., CA.

Children of JAMES BRUCKMAN and CLARA HILL are:

i. EDITH LOUISE BRUCKMAN (D71) was born on 20 Aug 1888 in CO and died 04 Oct 1980 in Orange Co., CA. She was never married. She is buried in Forest Lawn Memorial Park, Glendale, Los Angeles CO., CA.

ii. CLARA L. BRUCKMAN (D72) was born on 04 Nov 1890 in CO and died 17 Jan 1985 in Orange Co., CA. She was never married. She is buried in Forest Lawn Memorial Park, Glendale, Los Angeles CO., CA.

iii. ROBERT LESLIE BRUCKMAN (D73) was born in 07 Jul 1896 in CO and died 06 Feb 1986 in Marin Co., CA. He married ANNA ELIZABETH JASTROW on 30 Dec 1944 in Los Angeles, Los Angeles Co., CA, daughter of STEPHEN GRIFFITH JASTROW and SARAH SCOTT.

Ref: 29, 30, 8-Ward 1 Salt Lake City Salt lake Co UT F180, 33, 35, 26

D8 JOHN BRUCKMAN D

JOHN BRUCKMAN was born in Apr 1847 in New York City, New York Co., NY. He married SOPHIE KALISHER daughter of EDWARD DAVID KALISHER and BERTHA BETTY HERTZ. She was born in 25 Mar 1859 in Stockton, San Joaquin Co., CA and died 07 Mar 1950 in Ventura, Ventura Co., CA. She is buried in Cypress Lawn Memorial Park, Colma, San Mateo Co., CA.

Children of JOHN BRUCKMAN and SOPHIE KALISHER are:

i. HELEN BRUCKMAN, M.D. (D81) was born in 04 Dec 1890 in CA and died 15 Aug 1972 in CA. She is buried in Cypress Lawn Memorial Park, Colma, San Mateo Co., CA. She was a resident Pediatrician at University of California, San Francisco School of Medicine.

ii. BETTINA BRUCKMAN (D82) was born in Jul 1894 in CA and died 14 Nov 1986 in Contra Costra Co., CA. She is buried in Cypress Lawn Memorial Park, Colma, San Mateo Co., CA.

Ref: 8-San Francisco San Francisco Co CA F73, 33, 26

D9 FREDERICK BRUCKMAN D

FREDERICK BRUCKMAN was born in 1850 in New York City, New York Co., NY and died 1899 in Denver, Arapahoe Co., CO. He married REBECCA F. HALLOCK on 13 Apr 1880 in Arapahoe Co., CO, daughter of SAMUEL W. HALLOCK and CATHARINE FLAGLER. She was born in 1854 and died in 1896 in Denver, Arapahoe Co., CO. Both are buried in Fairmount Cemetery, Denver, Denver Co., CO.

Child of FREDERICK BRUCKMAN and REBECCA HALLOCK is:

   i. PHILIP S. BRUCKMAN (D91)

   ii. JOSEPHINE H. BRUCKMAN (D92)

   iii. HELEN T. BRUCKMAN (D93) was born in Sep 1884 in CO and died 19 Apr 1928 in Denver, Denver Co., CO. She is buried in Fairmount Cemetery, Denver, Denver Co., CO.

Ref: 29, 30, 8-Denver Arapahoe Co CO F132, 26

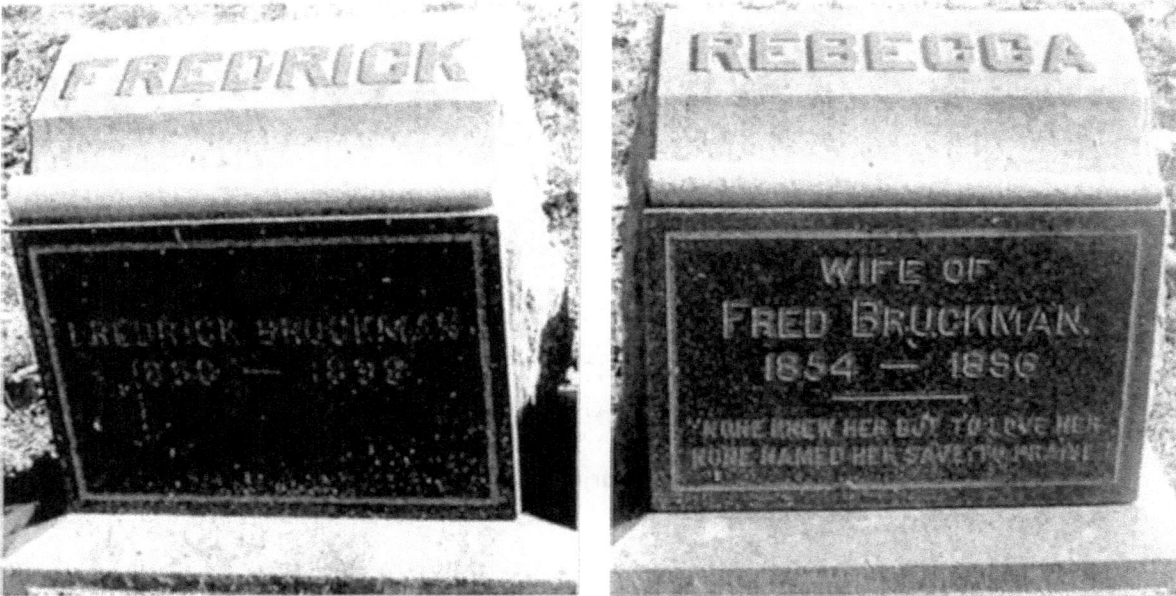

DA CHARLES BRUCKMAN D

CHARLES BRUCKMAN was born in May 1852 in New York City, New York Co., NY and died 1909 in Denver, Denver Co., CO. He married MARY TAUSSIG on 24 Sep 1885 in Denver, Arapahoe Co., CO. She was born in Sep 1856 in MO and died in 1929 in Denver, Denver Co., CO. Both are buried in Riverside Cemetery, Denver, Denver Co., CO

Children of CHARLES BRUCKMAN and MARY TAUSSIG are:

   i. CHARLES T. BRUCKMAN (DA1)

ii. FLORENCE L. BRUCKMAN (DA2) was born in May 1889 in CO. She married ROY W. ELLIOTT on 07 Sep 1935 in Colorado Springs, El Paso Co., CO.

Ref: 29, 26, 8-Denver Arapahoe Co CO F132, 10-Denver Denver Co CO F118, 9-Ward 10 Denver Denver Co CO F33

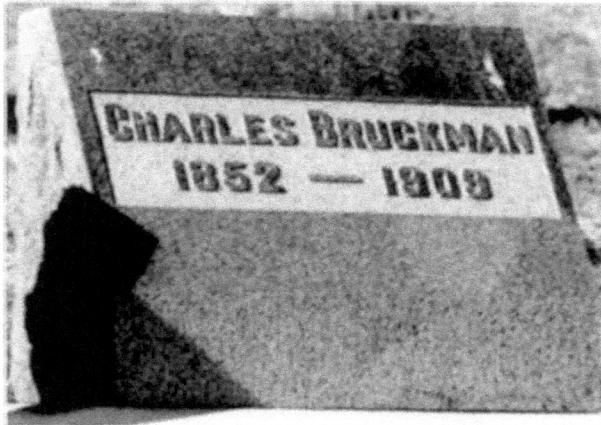

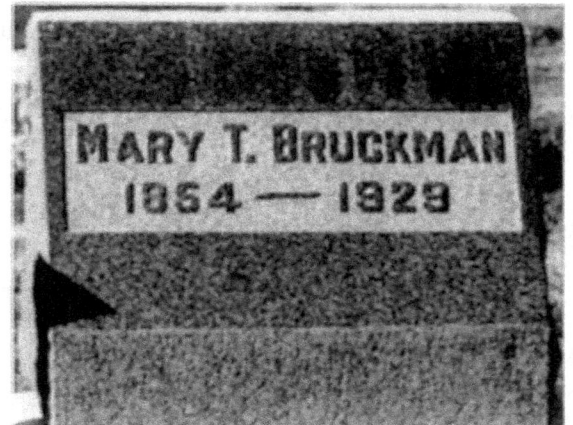

D51 GRACE HERMANITA BRUCKMAN D5

GRACE HERMANITA BRUCKMAN was born in 01 Aug 1883 in UT and died 20 Aug 1964 in Santa Clara Co., CA. She married HARRY HALL HOLLEY on 02 Jul 1906 in Santa Clara Co., CA, son of HILAND HOLLEY and MARY ELIZABETH SYKES. He was born on 16 Aug 1879 in Dorset, Co., Bennington Co., VT. GRACE HERMANITA BRUCKMAN, A.B., was Assistant in Physics, 1905-06, at Stanford University, CA. She was the first person in Visalia, CA to become a Baha'i in 1917 and practice this religious faith. He was a member of the Benevolent Protective Order of Elks, the American Society of Civil Engineers, the American Association of Engineers. Locally he was a member of the advisory council of the Sun Maid Raisin Growers Association, was a member of the city library board, member of the Delta Mosquito Abatement District, and of the local council of Boy Scouts. Besides his professional interests he was the owner of forty acres of fruit and vineyard near Ivanhoe.

Children of GRACE BRUCKMAN and HARRY HOLLEY are:

i. MARION H. HOLLEY (D511) was born on 17 May 1910 in Visalia, Tulare Co., CA and died 15 Dec 1995 in London, England. She married DAVID GEORGE RONALD HOFMAN in England. He was born on 23 Sep 1908 in Poona, India and died 09 May 2003 in England. She was a US track and field athlete who competed in the 1928 Summer Olympics and finished ninth in the high jump event. He served as a member of the Universal House of Justice, the supreme governing body of the Bahá'í Faith, between 1963 and 1988. He worked as the world's first television presenter for the British Broadcasting Corporation and later founded the publishing company George Ronald.

ii. SANFORD HOLLEY (D512) was born in 1914 in Visalia, Tulare Co., CA and died 07 Jan 1935 in Stockton, San Joaquin Co., CA. He was never married.

iii. RICHARD H. HOLLEY (D513) was born on 10 Oct 1915 in Visalia, Tulare Co., CA and died 01 Sep 1968 in Monterey Co., CA. He married HELEN _____ in CA. She was born in 1922 in CA.

iv. PATRICIA HOLLEY (D514) was born in 1917 in Visalia, Tulare Co., CA.

U.S. World War II Army Enlistment Records, 1938-1946
Name: Patricia Holley
Birth Year: 1917
Race: White, citizen (White)
State of Residence: California
County or City: Tulare
Enlistment Date: 19 Mar 1943
Enlistment State: California
Enlistment City: Los Angeles
Branch: Womens Army Corps
Branch Code: Inactive Reserve
Grade Code: Aviation Cadet
Term of Enlistment: Enlistment for the duration of the War or other emergency, plus six months, subject to the discretion of the President or otherwise according to law
Component: Womens Army Corps
Source: Civil Life
Education: 1 year of college
Civil Occupation: Telephone operators
Marital Status: Single, without dependents
Height: 78
Weight: 113

v. ANN HOLLEY (D515) was born in 1922 in Visalia, Tulare Co., CA.

Ref: 35, 34, 10-Visalia Tulare Co CA F50, 11-Visalia Tulare Co CA F186, 33, 55, 57-David_Hofman, 57-Marion_Holley, 58, 12-Fresno Fresno Co CA F256, 48

D91 PHILIP S. BRUCKMAN D9

PHILIP S. BRUCKMAN was born in Sep 1883 in CO and died 27 May 1933 in Denver, Denver Co., CO. He married FLOY E. ZINT on 15 Apr 1909 in Denver, Denver Co., CO, daughter of GEORGE W. ZINT and HATTIE J. _____ . She was born in 1881 and died in 1957 in Dayton, Montgomery Co., OH. He is buried in Fairmount Cemetery, Denver, Denver Co., CO. She is buried in Fairview Cemetery, Englewood, Montgomery Co., OH.

Child of PHILIP BRUCKMAN and FLOY ZINT is:

i. MELVIN E. BRUCKMAN (D911) was born in 31 Dec 1909 in Denver, Denver Co., CO and died Jul 1974 in CO.

Ref: 26, 9-Ward 14 Denver Denver Co CO H421, 10-Denver Denver Co CO F183, 42

JOSEPHINE H. BRUCKMAN was born in 30 Sep 1884 in CO and died 05 Jun 1927 in Moscow, Latah Co., ID. She married FRANCIS A. THOMPSON on 16 Aug 1906 in Golden, Jefferson Co., CO. She is buried in Odd Fellows Cemetery, Pullman, Whitman Co., WA.

Children of JOSEPHINE BRUCKMAN and are:

i. HELEN FRANCES THOMPSON (D921) was born in 1907 in Denver, Denver Co., CO. and died in 18 Dec 1910 in Denver, Denver Co., CO. She is buried in Odd Fellows Cemetery, Pullman, Whitman Co., WA.

ii. ANDREW H. THOMPSON (D922)

iii. ROBERT THOMPSON (D923) was born in 25 Dec 1911 in Denver, Denver Co., CO. and died in 04 Jan 1912 in Denver, Denver Co., CO. He is buried in Odd Fellows Cemetery, Pullman, Whitman Co., WA.

iv. RICHARD W. THOMPSON (D924) was born in 1915 in WA.

U.S. World War II Army Enlistment Records, 1938-1946
Name: Richard W Thomson
Birth Year: 1915
Race: White, citizen (White)
Nativity State or Country: Washington
State of Residence: New York
County or City: New York
Enlistment Date: 18 Apr 1941
Enlistment State: New York
Enlistment City: New York City
Branch: Branch Immaterial - Warrant Officers, USA
Branch Code: Branch Immaterial - Warrant Officers, USA
Grade: Private
Grade Code: Private
Component: Selectees (Enlisted Men)
Source: Civil Life
Education: 4 years of college
Civil Occupation: Clerks, general office
Marital Status: Single, without dependents
Height: 69
Weight: 129

Ref: 26, 31, 56, 9-Ward 3 Pullman Whitman Co WA F99, 10-Moscow Latah Co ID F20, 48

DA1 CHARLES T. BRUCKMAN DA

CHARLES T. BRUCKMAN was born on 30 Sep 1886 in CO and died in Feb 1974 in Denver, Denver Co., CO. He married LAURA C. COFFEY on 12 May 1909 in Denver, Denver Co., CO.

Children of CHARLES BRUCKMAN and LAURA COFFEY are:

  i. WILLIAM C. BRUCKMAN (DA11)

  ii. GEORGE HOYT BRUCKMAN (DA12)

  iii. KATHLEEN BRUCKMAN (DA13) was born in 1920 in Denver, Denver Co., CO. She married FRANKLIN JOSEPH MANNIX in CO, son of FRANKLIN JOSEPH MANNIX and ANNA LEE TOBIN. He was born on 15 Nov 1920 in CO and died 12 Dec 1970 in San Diego Co., CA.

Ref: 30, 9-Ward 10 Denver Denver Co CO F33, 10-Denver Denver Co CO F19, 11-Denver Denver Co CO F395, 42, 12-Denver Denver Co CO F232, 33

Wm. C. Bruckman's Mother Dies In Denver

William C. Bruckman, 1394 Pontiac road, received news this morning of the sudden death of his mother, Mrs. Charles T. Bruckman of Denver, Colo. during the night.

Mrs. Bruckman, who lived at 592 Franklin street, Denver, had been a patient in a hospital three weeks, although her death was sudden and unexpected.

Mr. Bruckman was to fly to Denver today to be with his family until after the funeral services. Funeral arrangements are incomplete.

Mrs. Bruckman is survived by her husband, her son in Benton Harbor, a son, George, of Denver, and a daughter, Mrs. Frank Mannix of San Diego, Calif. There are nine grandchildren.

The News Palladium 22 Apr 1957

D922 ANDREW H. THOMPSON D92

ANDREW H. THOMPSON was born in 1910 in Pullman, Whitman Co., WA. He married GRACE _____ in MT. She was born in 1910 in MT.

Children of ANDREW THOMPSON and GRACE _____ is:

i. RUTH J. THOMPSON (D9221) was born in 1939 in MT.

Ref: 12-Ward 2 Billings Yellowstone Co MT F211

DA11 WILLIAM C. BRUCKMAN DA1

WILLIAM C. BRUCKMAN was born in 1910 in Denver, Denver Co., CO and died 27 Apr 1960 in Los Angeles Co., CA. He married ELIZABETH G. GEIER in OH, daughter of _____ GEIER and _____ HORN. She was born in 21 Oct 1908 in OH and died 22 Dec 1990 in Los Angeles Co., CA.

Child of WILLIAM BRUCKMAN and ELIZABETH GEIER is:

i. RICHARD C. BRUCKMAN (DA111) was born in 1939 in OH.

Ref: 12-Ward 2 Mansfield Richland Co OH F279, 33

DA12 GEORGE HOYT BRUCKMAN DA1

GEORGE HOYT BRUCKMAN was born on 20 Nov 1912 in Denver, Denver Co., CO and died 16 Mar 2002. He married CLAIRE DALTON on 24 Oct 1936 Denver, Denver Co., CO. She was born in 10 Sep 1914 in OK and died on 01 Mar 1996 in Denver, Denver Co., CO.

Child of GEORGE BRUCKMAN and CLAIRE DALTON is:

i. CHARLES ELLIOTT BRUCKMAN (DA121)

ii. WALLACE DALE BRUCKMAN (DA122)

Ref: 12-Denver Denver Co CO F48, 30, 42

GEORGE H. BRUCKMAN, 89, of Denver died March 16. Services will be at 1 p.m. Monday, March 25, at Church of the Risen Christ Catholic Church. Mr. Bruckman was born in Denver on Nov. 20, 1912. He married Claire Dalton, 1936. He was a retired owner of an office products store. He was a member of the Lions Club, Denver Striker, Rocky Mountain Striker and Knights of Columbus. Survivors include sons Charles of Bailey, Dal of Evergreen; five grandchildren; five great-grandchildren.

Rocky Mountain News 25 March 2002

DA121 CHARLES ELLIOTT BRUCKMAN DA12

CHARLES ELLIOTT BRUCKMAN was born on 20 Dec 1938 in Denver, Denver Co., CO. He married SHARLENE "SHARON" M. OWEN in CO. She was born on 11 Sep 1941.

Children of CHARLES BRUCKMAN and SHARLENE OWEN are:

i. STEVEN E. BRUCKMAN (DA1211) was born on 09 Feb 1966 in CO.

ii. STUART LEWIS BRUCKMAN (DA1212) was born on 09 Oct 1969 in CO.

Ref: 49

DA122 WALLACE DALE BRUCKMAN DA12

WALLACE DALE BRUCKMAN was born on 08 Apr 1941 in Denver, Denver Co., CO. He married CAROL HILL DURGIN in CO. She was born on 26 Dec 1945.

Children of WALLACE BRUCKMAN and CAROL DURGIN are:

i. DANIEL E. BRUCKMAN (DA1221) was born on 22 Jul 1972

ii. JULIE LYNN BRUCKMAN (DA1222) was born on 30 Nov 1974

Ref: 49

CHAPTER 6

E JACOB GEORGE BRUCKMAN II

Dr. JACOB GEORGE BRUCKMAN was born on 27 Mar 1800 in House #11, Loschitz, Bohemia, Austria (now Loštice, Czech Republic) and died 10 Dec 1885 in Clearville, Bedford Co., PA. He is buried in Bedford Cemetery on route 220, Bedford Co., PA. He married SARAH LINDEMAN in Somerset Co., PA, daughter of JACOB LINDEMAN and ELIZABETH NICHOLSON. She was born 07 Jun 1810 in Somerset Co., PA, and died 26 Jul 1861 in Salisbury, Somerset Co., PA. She is buried at *Salisbury Old Cemetery*, Salisbury, Somerset Co., PA. His arrival in America is now believed to be around the same time in 1842 as his brother, both arriving at the port of New York City. The correct passenger list has yet to be found and quite possibly has been destroyed or lost. There are records of other BRUCKMANs arriving that year but their given names remain a mystery. He filed a *declaration of intention* to become a United States naturalized citizen recorded at Somerset County Courthouse, Somerset, PA, during the December 1842 term, as a copy of that court record included attests.

Although the naturalization declaration record states he is a native of Austria. In the 1880 census his place of birth is given as Bohemia. At that time in history Bohemia was ruled by the Austro-Hungarian Empire monarchy so Bohemia and/or Austria would have been correct at that period of time. Firstly, that the census enumeration was completed by his son-in-law, Dr. AMERICUS ENFIELD. Secondly Dr. Enfield, acting as the census taker, appears when looking at the actual census record made a concerted effort to correct and change his father-in-law's place of birth from Austria to Bohemia, reason unknown.

Dr. JACOB GEORGE BRUCKMAN was a physician by occupation. It is said and written that he studied at the University of Prague for about seven years and graduated there in 1831 as a Doctor of Medicine. In the attempt to discover his exact birthplace has manifested some serious questions regarding his alleged attendance and graduation from the University of Prague. The author has been in contact with PH. Dr. ZDENEK POUSTA of the Institute for the History of Charles University, Archive of Charles University, Prague, Czechoslovakia (now Czech Republic). Dr. POUSTA and others have conducted a search of the student lists of the medical facility and the register of doctors at the facility from 1831 to 1840 with negative results. Dr. POUSTA then suggested that I make inquiry to the University in Vienna. I made contact with the Dr. KURT MÜHLBERGER of University of Wien (Vienne) and archivist PETER GOLLER of the University of Innsbruck. JACOB GEORGE BRUCKMAN was not found in the records of the University of Wien (Vienna) from 1821 to 1841 without success and the University of Innsbruck did not have an active medical facility from 1810 to 1869. In addition ALEXANDRA JAHN, University Library of Innsbruck conducted a search of the microfiche edition of the *German Biographical Archive* without success either. The University of Graz in Austria has also been ruled out, as a possible place of study as is did not have an active medical facility during the time period in question. Based on recent research discoveries the Palacký University located in Olomouc and the second-oldest in the Czech Republic has come to be the most likely place of study for Dr. JACOB GEORGE BRUCKMAN. It is located not far to the southeast of Loschitz where he was born. This university was established in 1573 as a public university led by the Jesuit order in Olomouc, which at that time the capital of Moravia and the seat of the episcopacy. At first it taught only theology, but soon the fields of philosophy, law and medicine were added. It was active for medical studies about 1827-1831 when Dr. JACOB GEORGE BRUCKMAN would have completed his studies.

The author recently contacted, CHARLES ENFIELD MCDERMOTT, a descendant through daughter, MARY REBECCA BRUCKMAN, who married AMERICUS ENFIELD. It is through this correspondence that the author learned the Dr. JACOB GEORGE BRUCKMAN's original Austrian medical practice certificate/license was in the possession of CHARLES ENFIELD MCDERMOTT. This document was passed down through several generations to him by his mother when she died in 1985. A copy of this document serves as definitive proof of the author's research determining Dr. JACOB GEORGE BRUCKMAN's birth place and parentage. A copy of this document is provided and clearly indicates his birth place as Loschitz (in German) (now Loštice, Czech Republic). It also indicates he stated his medical practice in 1831 and says he completed his medical board exams in Prag, Böhmen, Austria (now Prague/Praha, Czech Republic. Prague is the historical capital of Bohemia. It is the author's assumption that those who have wrote about Dr. JACOB GEORGE BRUCKMAN in the past that may have seen certificate may have mistaken the place of board exams as the place he had gone to school. The certificate makes no mention of where he attended medical school.

Based on recent information supplied to the author from a cousin, WILLIAM RICHARD GRIFFITH, it is reasonable to assume that Dr. JACOB GEORGE BRUCKMAN was in all likelihood a Böhmen Jew when he arrived in America. Given that Jews were at this time in the mid 19th century were believe to be inferior were often mistreated and suffered inhumane restrictions placed on them to limit their very existence. One of those restrictions for a period of time was that the only the oldest living male child of a Jewish family was allowed to married and have children. The only way another male child could marry would only be allowed if the older child was deceased. That being said many Jews at that period of time fled this unjust persecution to other more favorable lands, one of which was America. It is certain Dr. JACOB GEORGE BRUCKMAN and his brother Dr. PHILIP BRUCKMAN both came to American for that reason. The aforementioned male marriage restriction is certainly why Dr. JACOB GEORGE BRUCKMAN was not yet married at such an elevated age when he arrived in America, since his brother was older than him and married when he arrived. It is believed over time the details of his professional achievements and development as a physician became victim to stretching the facts for a greater human interest as do most all family histories to some degree. The author has yet to discover if Dr. JACOB GEORGE BRUCKMAN ever practiced his Jewish faith after arrival in America, assumably to ensure he and his future family did not experience or subject themselves to long lived oppression he had previously endured.

Children of JACOB BRUCKMAN and SARAH LINDEMAN are:

i. ELIZABETH BRUCKMAN (E1) born on 07 Jun 1845 in Salisbury, Somerset Co., PA and died 04 May 1856, Salisbury, Somerset Co., PA. She never married and is buried at Old Salisbury Cemetery, Salisbury, Somerset Co., PA.

ii. MARY REBECCA BRUCKMAN (E2)

iii. FRANKLIN DAVID BRUCKMAN (E3)

iv. MARTHA JANE BRUCKMAN (E4)

Ref: 1, 8-Bedford Borough Bedford Co PA, 4-Elklick Twp Somerset Co PA, 5-Elklick Twp Somerset Co PA, 6-Elklick Twp Somerset Co PA, 7-Clearville Bedford Co PA, 3, 2, 22, 36, 67, 68

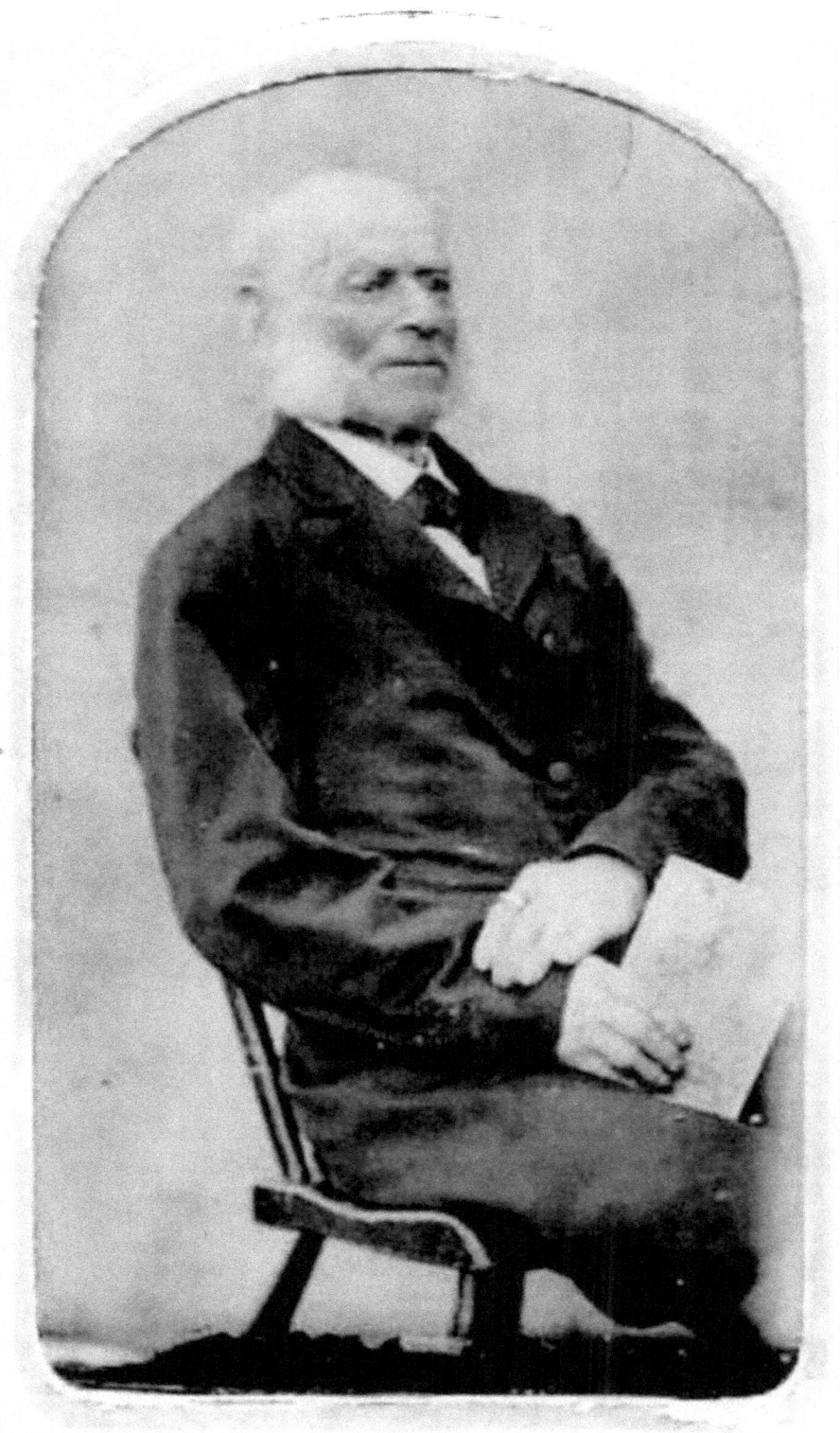

Dr. JACOB GEORGE BRUCKMAN

WIR VORSTEHER DES CHIRURGISCHEN GREMIUMS

des _____ lich es bekennen hiemit, daß nachdem der Herr Wundarzt _____

geburtig von _____ in _____ die Dokumente vorgebrachter Ausbildung laut dem Zeugnisse über die Prüfungen aus der Chirurgie und Geburtshilfe zu _____ in _____ den _____ im Jahr 18__ dann die Befugniß zur Ausübung der Praxis-Ausübung nachweislich in _____ _____ In diesem ihm vorschriftsmäßig nachgewiesen hat, Wir keinen Anstand nehmen, denselben als _____ Mitglied unserm chirurgischen Gremium gehörig einzutreten.

_____

So geschehen bei dem _____ chirurgischen Kreisgremium zu _____

_____ den _____ im Jahre 18__

Coram me _____

Dr. JACOB GEORGE BRUCKMAN 1st license to practice medicine
(In the possession of descendant Charles Enfield McDermott on October 23, 2014)

License Translation
We, the Principals of the Surgical Board
of the *Pilsner* (Pilsen District/Czechia) district, herewith declare that the surgeon, Mr. *Jakob Brückman*, born in *Loschitz* (Loštice) in *Mähren* (Moravia/Czechia) has furnished – according to regulations – the documents of lawful qualification in conformity with the certificate of examinations in surgery and obstetrics at *Prag* (Prague) in *Böhmen* (Bohemia) from the *13th of December to the 18th of June* in the year *1831*. He has also earned the authority for establishment and practice specifically in *Brennporitschen* (Spálené Poříčí/ Czechia) in this district. We do not hesitate to accept the aforementioned surgeon as a Board Member into our Surgical Board.
The proper admission of the surgeon *Jakob G. Brückman* valid and, in case he decides to move to another district, he is obliged to duly report his transfer to the Board, and the board members shall entitle him to practice under the terms of Paragraph 19 of the Board Decree dated *November 18, 1822*.
In verification of this we have the certificate personally signed not only but also sealed with the seal of the board.
This took place at the *Pilsener* (Pilsen District) Surgical Board at *Pilsen* on *July 4th* in the year *1831*.

The presence of   *Joseph Reis*
Dr. Tuscher   *district surgeon as head*
district physician   *of the surgical council*
as General-Board   *J. Habenicht second head*

JACOB GEORGE BRUCKMAN birth record

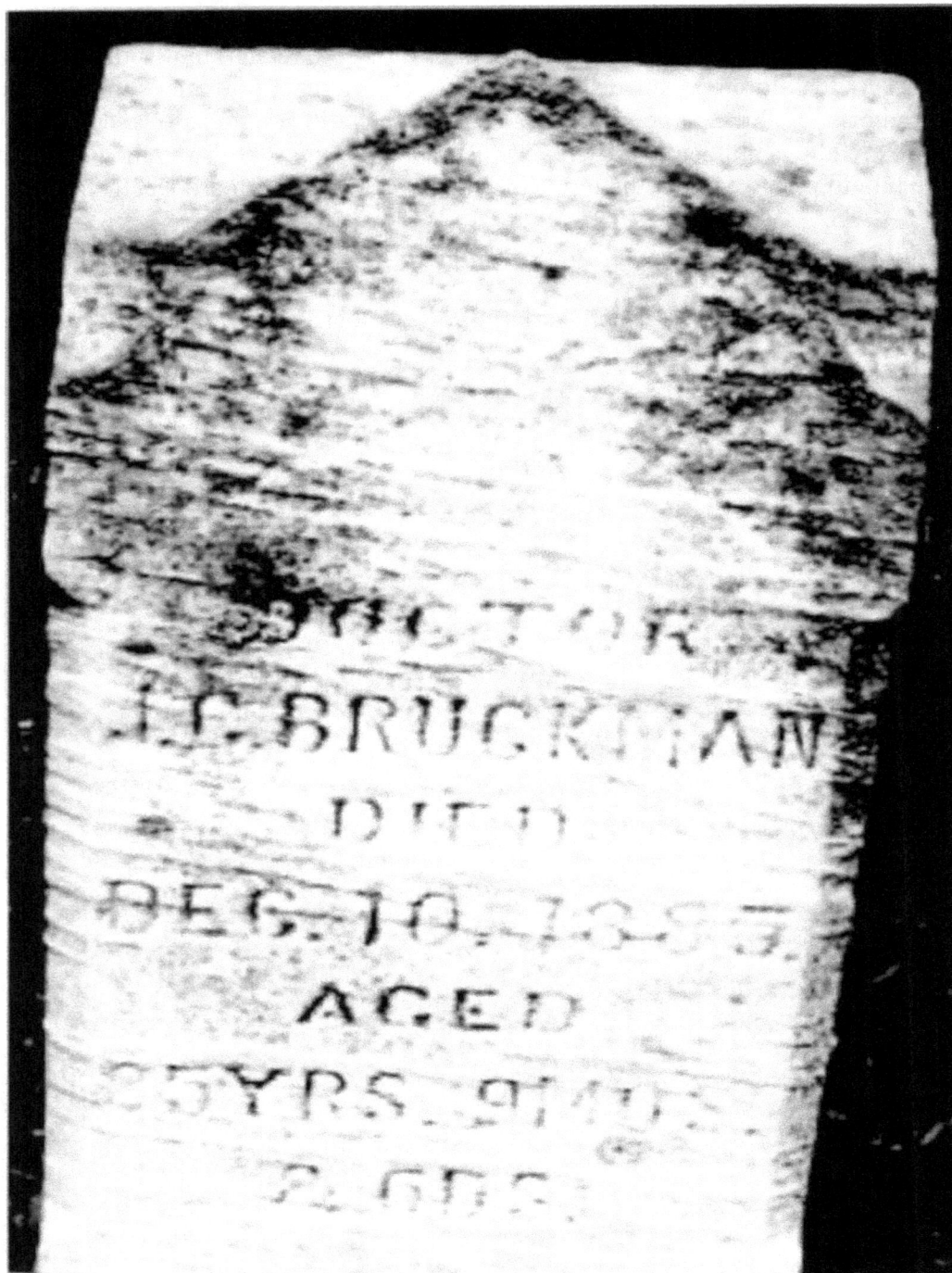

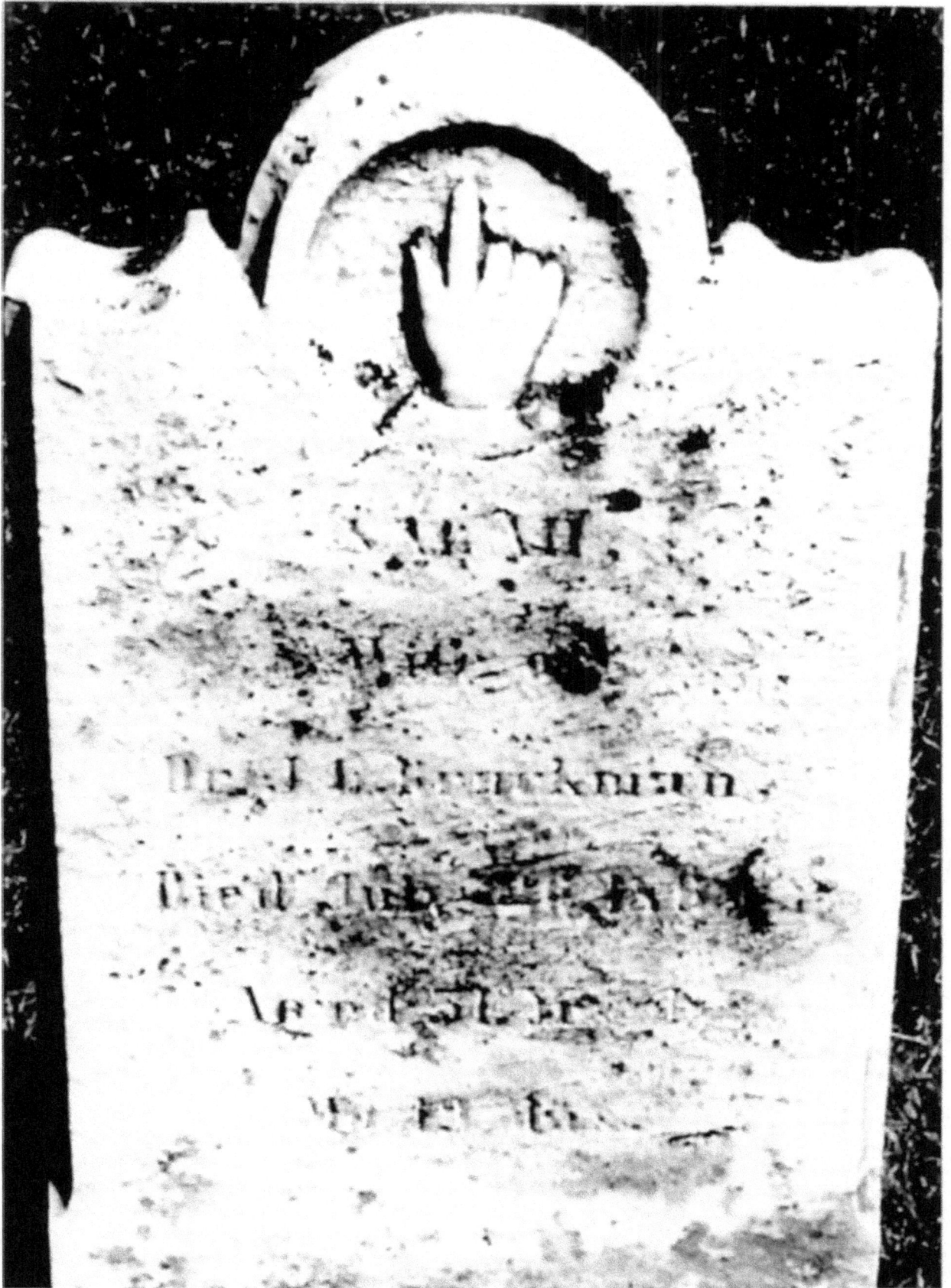

SARAH (LINDEMAN) BRUCKMAN

D E E D   } This Indenture made the twenty fourth day of November
M M. Miller   } in the year of our Lord one thousand eight hundred and
wife   }   fifty six (1856) Between Moses M. Miller of Elklick Township
         } Somerset County and State of Pennsylvania & Catharine his wife
J. G. Brookman's parties of the first part and Jacob G. Brookman of the Town of
Salisbury Township County and State aforesaid party of the second
part Witnesseth that the said parties of the first part for and in consideration of the sum of Sixty dollars lawful money of the United
States of America unto them well and truly paid by the said
party of the second part at or before the sealing and delivery of these
presents the receipt whereof is hereby acknowledged have granted bargained
sold aliened enfeoffed released conveyed and confirmed and by these
presents do grant bargain sell alien enfeoff release convey and
confirm unto the said party of the second part his heirs and assigns
All the following described lot piece or parcel of land situate in
Elklick Township Somerset County Commonwealth of Pennsylvania
bounded as follows— Beginning at stones thence by lot of said
J. G. Brookman south nineteen degrees & a half west sixteen perches
and one tenth to a post thence by lands of Samuel Wolfelsberger south
sixty four degrees east twenty perches to a post thence by the original
and lands of Moses M. Miller south nineteen degrees & a half east
sixteen perches & one tenth perches thence by the same north sixty
four degrees west twenty perches to the place of beginning Containing
two acres strict measure being part of a larger tract of land
which was conveyed to Moses M. Miller by deed the 26th of April
A.D. 1856 by Peter Livengood wife to the said Moses M. Miller the
present grantor reference to said titles being had more fully and
at large Appears— Together with all and singular the improvements
ways waters water courses rights liberties privileges hereditaments
and appurtenances whatsoever thereunto belonging or in anywise
appertaining and the reversions and remainders rents issues
and profits thereof And all the estate right title interest
property claim and demand whatsoever of the said parties of
the first part of in law equity or otherwise howsoever of in and
to the same and every part thereof To have and to hold
the said piece or parcel of land hereditaments & premises
hereby granted or mentioned and intended so to be with the
appurtenances unto the said party of the second part his heirs
and assigns to and for the only proper use and behoof of the said
party of the second part his heirs and assigns forever And
Moses M. Miller and wife the said parties of the first part
their heirs all and singular the hereditaments and premises
Executors and administrators as by these presents covenant
grant and agree to and with the said party of the second part his
heirs & assigns that they the said parties of the first part &
their heirs all and singular the hereditaments & premises herein
above described and granted or mentioned and intended
so to be with the appurtenances unto the said party of

the second part his heirs and assigns, against them the said
parties of the first part and their heirs and against all and every
other person or persons whomsoever lawfully claiming or to
claim the same or any part thereof shall & will warrant
and forever defend.

In witness whereof the said parties of the first
part have to these presents set their hands & seals, dated the
day and year first above written.

Sealed & delivered in the
presence of us C. G. Stutzman
        Hezekiah Haun

Moses W. Miller
Cattarine ☩ Miller
            mark

Recd the day of the date of the above Indenture of the
above named Jacob G. Brookman the sum of sixty
(60) dollars the consideration money above mentioned in full
C. G. Stutzman   Moses W. Miller
Hezekiah Haun

Somerset County ss.

On the 24 of November Anno Domini 1856, before
me a Justice of the Peace came the above named Moses W. Miller
and Cattarine his wife and acknowledged the above Indenture
to be their act and deed, and desired the same might be
recorded as such. She the said Cattarine Miller being of
lawful age and separate and apart from her said husband
by me examined and the contents of the said Indenture being first
made fully known to her declared that she did of her own
free will and accord sign and seal and as her act and deed
delivers the same without any coercion or compulsion of
her said husband.

Jas. G. Stutzman
            J. Pee

Recorded the 14th of October 1869
                    Aug. Davis
                        Recorder

William S. Lichty
&
J. G. Bruckman

This Indenture, made the second day of April in the year of our Lord one thousand eight hundred and Seventy. Between William S. Lichty and wife his wife of Salisbury Borough of the first part, and J. G. Bruckman of the same place of the second part. Witnesseth, That the said parties of the first part, for and in consideration of the sum of Fifteen Hundred Dollars, lawful money of the United States of America unto them well and truly paid by the said party of the second part, at or before the sealing and delivery of these presents, the receipt whereof is hereby acknowledged, have granted, bargained, sold, aliened, enfeoffed, released, conveyed and confirmed, and by these presents do grant, bargain, sell, alien, enfeoff, release, convey and confirm unto the said party of the second part, his heirs and assigns. All the following described lot of ground in the Borough of Salisbury marked No. 4 on the original plot of said town. Bounded on the North by Union Street on the West by — Street on the South by a lot now owned by Aug. Rosenberger being the same lately conveyed by William Smith & wife to the present grantor. Together with all and singular the buildings, improvements, ways, waters, water courses, rights, liberties, privileges, hereditaments and appurtenances, whatsoever thereunto belonging or in any wise appertaining, and the reversions and remainders, rents, issues, and profits thereof; and all the estate, right, title, interest, property, claim and demand whatsoever of the said parties of the first part, in law, equity, or otherwise howsoever of, in and to the same and every part thereof.

To have and to hold the said lot of ground, buildings, hereditaments and premises hereby granted or mentioned, and intended so to be, with the appurtenances, unto the said party of the second part, his heirs and assigns, to and for the only proper use and behoof of the said party of the second part, his heirs and assigns, forever. And William S. Lichty & wife the said parties of the first part, their heirs, executors and administrators, do, by these presents, covenant, grant, and agree to and with the said party of the second part, his heirs and assigns, that they, the said parties of the first part, their heirs, all and singular the hereditaments and premises hereinabove described and granted or mentioned, and intended so to be, with the appurtenances, unto the said party of the second part, his heirs and assigns, against them the said parties of the first part, and their heirs, and against all and every other person or persons whomsoever lawfully claiming or to claim the same or any part thereof. Shall and will warrant and forever defend. In witness whereof, the said parties of the first part, have to these presents set their hands and seals.___ Dated the day and year first above written.

Sealed and Delivered
in the presence of us:
Sam Hier
Samuel J. Lichty

William S. Lichty [seal]

Sadie E. Lichty [seal]

U.S.I.R.S.
50 cents

Received the day of the date of the above Indenture, of the above named Dr. J. G. Bruckman the sum of Fifteen Hundred Dollars, lawful money of the United States, being the consideration money above mentioned, in full.

U.S.I.R.S.
50 cents

Witness:
Sam Hier

Wm. S. Lichty

Somerset County, ss:
On the 2ⁿ day of April Anno Domini 1870, before me, a Justice of the Peace in & for said County, came the above named William C. Lichty and Sadie his wife, and acknowledged the above Indenture; to be their act and deed, and desired that the same might be recorded as such. She, the said Sadie being of full age, and by me examined separate and apart from her said husband, and the contents of the said Indenture being first made fully known to her, declared that she did, of her own free will and accord, sign and seal, and as her act and deed deliver the same without any coercion or compulsion of her said husband.
Witness my hand and seal the day and year aforesaid.

Recorded 2ⁿ April 1891.   Sam Weir J.P.

A.J. Hileman
Recorder

E2 MARY REBECCA BRUCKMAN E

MARY REBECCA BRUCKMAN was born in Dec 1846, Salisbury, Somerset Co., PA and died 19 Jan 1919 in Bedford, Bedford Co., PA. She married Dr. AMERICUS ENFIELD on 01 Aug 1870 in Salisbury, Somerset Co., PA. He was born on 07 Apr 1847, Salisbury, Somerset Co., PA and died 02 Apr 1931, Bedford, Bedford Co., PA. Both are buried in Bedford Cemetery on route 220, Bedford Co., PA. He served in the Civil War from PA as a Private in the Ringgold Battalion of Cavalry, Company G. He was a physician by occupation & served as Bedford County Sheriff. He left a will record in Book 15, Page 108 Bedford County Courthouse, Bedford, Bedford Co., PA.

Children of MARY BRUCKMAN and AMERICUS ENFIELD are:

i. WALTER F. ENFIELD (E21)

ii. FANNIE Z. ENFIELD (E22) was born on 02 Feb 1875 in Elk Lick, Somerset Co., PA and died 17 Jan 1956 in Harrison Twp., Bedford Co., PA. She was never married.

iii. CHARLES L. ENFIELD (E23)

iv. OLIVE MAY ENFIELD (E24) was born on 29 Jan 1877in Clearville, Bedford Co., PA and died 30 Mar 1961 in Harrison Twp., Bedford Co., PA. She was never married.

v. MILTON H. S. ENFIELD (E25) was born on 09 Jul 1879 in Bedford Co., PA and died 22 Oct 1933 in Bedford, Bedford Co., PA. He was never married.

vi. MARY REBECCA ENFIELD (E26) was born in Mar 1884 in Bedford Co., PA. She married HUGH H. LEGGE. He was born in 1885 in IL.

Mr. and Mrs. H. H. Legge of Cresson spent Christmas with the latter's sisters. Misses Fannie and Olive Enfield.

The Bedford Gazette 31 Dec 1946

Mrs. H. H. Legge of Cresson is visiting her sister Miss Fannie Enfield.

The Bedford Gazette 22 May 1947

Ref: 36, 26, 7-Bedford Bedford Co PA F266, 8-Clearville Bedford Co PA F121, 27-D-MHSE-86176, 27-DFZE-1835, 11-Los Angeles Los Angeles Co CA F165

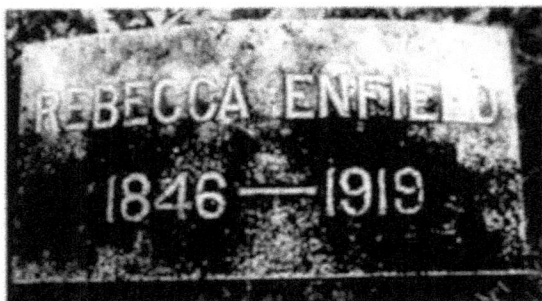

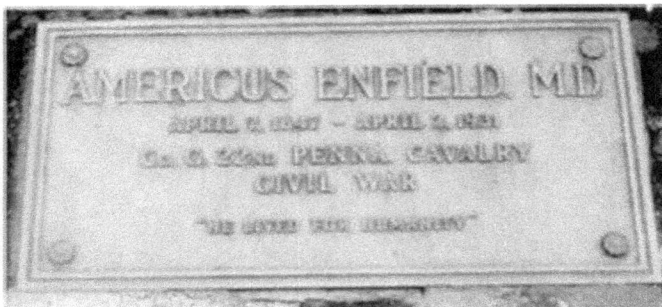

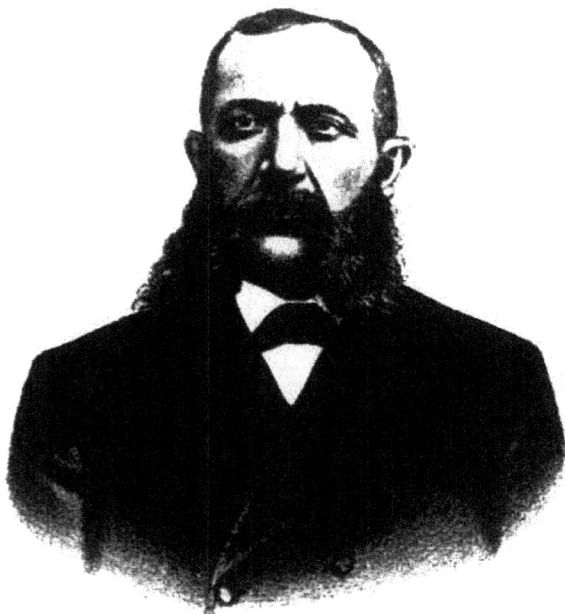

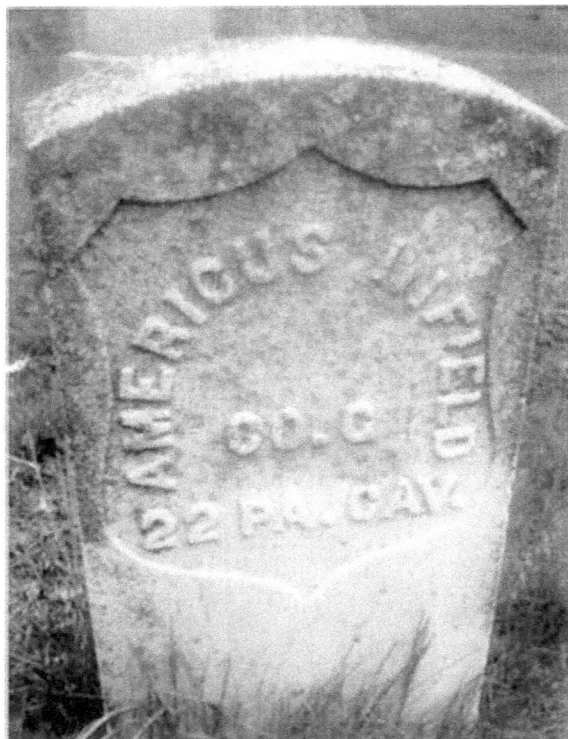

ESTIMABLE WIFE AND MOTHER

Who had a Host of Friends Passes Away

The death of Mrs. Rebecca Enfield occurred at her home Penn and Thomas streets, Bedford at six o'clock Sunday morning January 19, 1919, after an illness of two months.

Mrs. Enfield was aged 72 years and was the daughter of the late Dr. J. G. Bruckman of Somerset County. On August 1, 1870 she was united in marriage to Dr. Americus Enfield, now Postmaster of Bedford who with the following children survive: Dr. Walter F. Milton S, Fannie, Olive and Mary of this place sister, Mrs. Martha De Losier of Salisbury, also survives.

The home, the church and the reparable loss in the death of Mrs. Enfield who was a devoted wife and mother. Her kind words and deeds will long be remembered by a host of true friends.

The funeral services were held from her late home, Wednesday afternoon at 2 o'clock, conducted by Lutheran Church of which the deceased was a faithful member. Rev Allenbach was assisted by Rev. Eyler of the Reformed Church and Rev. Bell of the Methodist church.

Interment was made in the Bedford cemetery.

Altoona Mirror 21 May 1969

Americus Enfield Dead at Bedford
Aged Physician and Politician Passed Away After Long and Useful Career

Dr. Americus Enfield, aged 84, who for half a century was a familiar figure in Bedford County medical and political circles, passed away last Thursday night at 9 o'clock, following an illness of several weeks. Dr. Enfield was born in 1847, in Elk Lick Township, Somerset County, where his ancestors settled shortly after the Revolutionary War. The Enfield family came to this country before the Revolutionary War and for many years manufactured rifles in the New England States. The family was engaged in the manufacture of firearms in England for many years. Enfield, England, was named after the Enfield family, and is the seat of the well-known government manufactory of rifles and small arms and the standard rifle, used in the British army, also is made there. The original Enfield rifle was a muzzleloading rifle and was used in the British army prior to the introduction of the breech-loading system. It also was used in the United States during the Civil War by the Northern Army, when Springfield rifles could not be obtained. Some Enfield rifles also were used by the Confederate Army. In England large numbers of the Enfield rifles were converted into breechloaders on the Snider principle and were then known as the Snider-Enfield rifles. Dr. Enfield was the proud possessor of the first Enfield rifle manufactured in America. He received his early education in the public schools at Salisbury, and later the Academy at Somerset. Soon after the outbreak of the Civil War, Dr. Enfield entered the artillery service and participated in the battle of Gettysburg, where he was wounded. Following his recovery he enlisted in the U.S. Cavalry, in which service he remained until October 31, 1865. Dr. Enfield taught school in West Virginia for two years and later entered Mercersburg, (Pa.) College. He then went to the office of Dr. G. B. Fundenburg, an ex-army surgeon, in Cumberland, Md., where he remained for two years studying medicine and then entered Jefferson Medical College, Philadelphia, and later Bellevue Medical College and Hospital in New York City. After his graduation from that institution, he practiced in Cumberland and later at Flintstone, Md. In 1870 he located at Clearville, Bedford County, Pa., as a medical practitioner. A few years later he was elected Sheriff of Bedford County and moved to Bedford, where he had since resided. An ardent Democrat, Dr. Enfield was one of the most active and best known Democratic politicians in Pennsylvania for more than half a century. He was a delegate to nearly every Democratic National Convention since the Civil War. He was acting chairman during part of the sessions of the convention in Baltimore in 1912, which resulted in the nomination for Woodrow Wilson for President. He was postmaster of Bedford for nine years by appointment by President Wilson. On several occasions he was a candidate for

Congress in the old Cambria-Blair-Bedford district. Last year he was the unsuccessful Democratic candidate for State Senator in the Somerset-Bedford-Fulton district, being defeated by Hon. Charles H. Ealy, of Somerset, a native of Bedford County. During most of his life Dr. Enfield wore flowing sidewiskers. He was a fine-looking man and picturesque character of kind and generous disposition. Having spent his boyhood along the banks of Piney Run in Elk Lick Township, Dr. Enfield became an expert trout fisher, and during his old age he loved to return each spring to his native heath to fish for trout in Piney Run. Dr. Enfield's wife, who was Miss Rebecca Bruckman, of Salisbury, died some years ago. The following children survive: Dr. Walter F. Enfield, the Misses Fannie and Olive, and Milton S. Enfield, all of Bedford; Charles Enfield, of McKeesport, and Mrs. Mary Legge, of Los Angeles, Cal. Of his five grandchildren, two are physicians, Dr. Thomas Enfield, of Philadelphia, and Dr. George S. Enfield, of Bedford. Funeral services were conducted Sunday afternoon at his late home and were largely attended. Rev. J. Albert Eyler, pastor of the Bedford Reformed Church, officiated. Interment was in the Bedford Cemetery.

Meyersdale Republican 09 Apr 1931

DEED
J. G. Brockman
To
Rebecca Enfield

This Indenture Made the ninth day of November in the year of our Lord one thousand eight hundred and seventy six: Between Dr J. G. Brockman of the Borough of Salisbury in the County of Somerset and State of Pennsylvania of the first part and Rebecca Brockman now intermarried with Dr Americus Enfield of the County of Bedford and State aforesaid of the second part Witnesseth that the said party of the first part for and in consideration of the sum of one dollar and natural love and affection for his said daughter Rebecca lawful money of the United States of America unto him well and truly paid by the said party of the second part at and before the executing and delivery of these presents the receipt whereof is hereby acknowledged has granted bargained sold aliened enfeoffed released conveyed and confirmed and by these presents doth grant bargain sell alien enfeoff release convey and confirm unto the said party of the second part her heirs and assigns,

All the following described Lot of ground situate in the Borough of Salisbury in the County of Somerset and State aforesaid marked as Lot No 4 on the original plan of said Borough bounded on the north by Union Street on the west by Bay Street on the south by a Lot now owned by Long Rosenberger It being the same premises which were conveyed by William I Lichty and wife to grantor by deed bearing date the 2nd day of April AD 1870

Together with all and singular the buildings improvements woods ways rights liberties privileges hereditaments and appurtenances to the same belonging or in anywise appertaining and the reversion and reversions remainder and remainders rents issues and profits thereof and of every part and parcel thereof And also all the estate right title interest property possession claim and demand whatsoever both in law and equity of the said party of the first part of in and to the said premises with the appurtenances To have and to hold the said premises with all and singular the appurtenances unto the said party of the second part her heirs and assigns to the only proper use benefit and behoof of the said party of the second part her heirs and assigns forever

And J. G. Brockman the said party of the first part his heirs executors and administrators do by these presents covenant grant and agree to and with the said party of the second part her heirs and assigns that he the said J. G. Brockman his heirs all and singular the hereditaments and premises herein above described and granted or mentioned and intended to be so with the appurtenances unto the said party of the second part her heirs and assigns against them the said J. G. Brockman his heirs and against all and every other person or persons whomsoever lawfully claiming or to claim the same or any part thereof by from or under them or any of them Shall and will warrant and forever defend

In witness whereof the said party of the first part to these presents hereunto set his hand and seal Dated the day and year first above written.

Signed sealed and delivered
In the presence of
David P Maus
William Trimer

J. G. Brockman [seal]

E3 FRANKLIN DAVID BRUCKMAN E

FRANKLIN DAVID BRUCKMAN was born 27 Jun 1849 in Salisbury, Somerset Co., PA, and died 03 Nov 1899 in Harrisburg, Dauphin Co., PA. He married MARY EMMA RITCHEY about 1879 in Bedford Co., PA, daughter of PHILIP R. RITCHEY and MARY EMMA MIKESELL. She was born 18 Oct 1862 in Everett, Bedford Co., PA, and died 03 Sep 1923 in Altoona, Blair Co., PA. Both are buried at Everett Cemetery, Bedford Co., PA. He was a teacher and carpenter by occupation. He was employed as an IRS Agent living in Schellsburg, Bedford, PA on 01 Jul1889. Six of the children were baptized on 05 Apr 1890 at St. John's United Church of Christ (formerly St. John's Evangelical & Reformed Church) Bedford, Bedford Co., PA by Rev. R. L. Gerhart.

Children of FRANKLIN BRUCKMAN and MARY RITCHEY are:

i. MARY REBECCA BRUCKMAN (E31)

ii. ANNA ELIZABETH BRUCKMAN (E32)

iii. HARRY VINCENT BRUCKMAN (E33)

iv. ALICE MAY BRUCKMAN (E34)

v. CHARLES HERBERT BRUCKMAN (E35)

vi. FANNIE ZELUMA BRUCKMAN (E36)

vii. ARTHUR FRANKLIN BRUCKMAN (E37)

viii. JOHN ELLIS BRUCKMAN (E38)

Ref: 2, 12-Monroe Twp Bedford Co PA, 12-Altoona Blair Co PA, 8-Everett Borough Bedford Co PA, 7-West Providence Twp Bedford Co PA, 13-Monroe Twp, 10-823 2nd Avenue Altoona Blair Co PA, 10-Greenfield Twp Blair Co PA, 10-Logan Twp Blair Co PA, 8-Elklick Twp Somerset Co PA; 21

REGISTER OF BAPTISMS.

51

No.	NAME OF SUBJECT.	No.	BORN.	WHEN BAPTIZED.	INFANT.	ADULT.	BY WHOM BAPTIZED.
	Harry Hafer Bolinger		sept 5th 88	June 23 89	1		R. L. Gerhart
	N... M... D...		...	...			"
	Fannie Zeloma Brockman		March 11 89	April 5 90	1		" " "
	Charles Herbert Brockman		Aug 21 87	" " "	1		" " "
	Alice May Brockman		Jan 11 85	" " "	1		" " "
	Harry Vincent Brockman		Oct 23 83	" " "	1		" " "
	Annie Lizzie Brockman		March 2 82	" " "	1		" " "
	Mary Rebecca Brockman		March 15 81	" " "	1		" " "

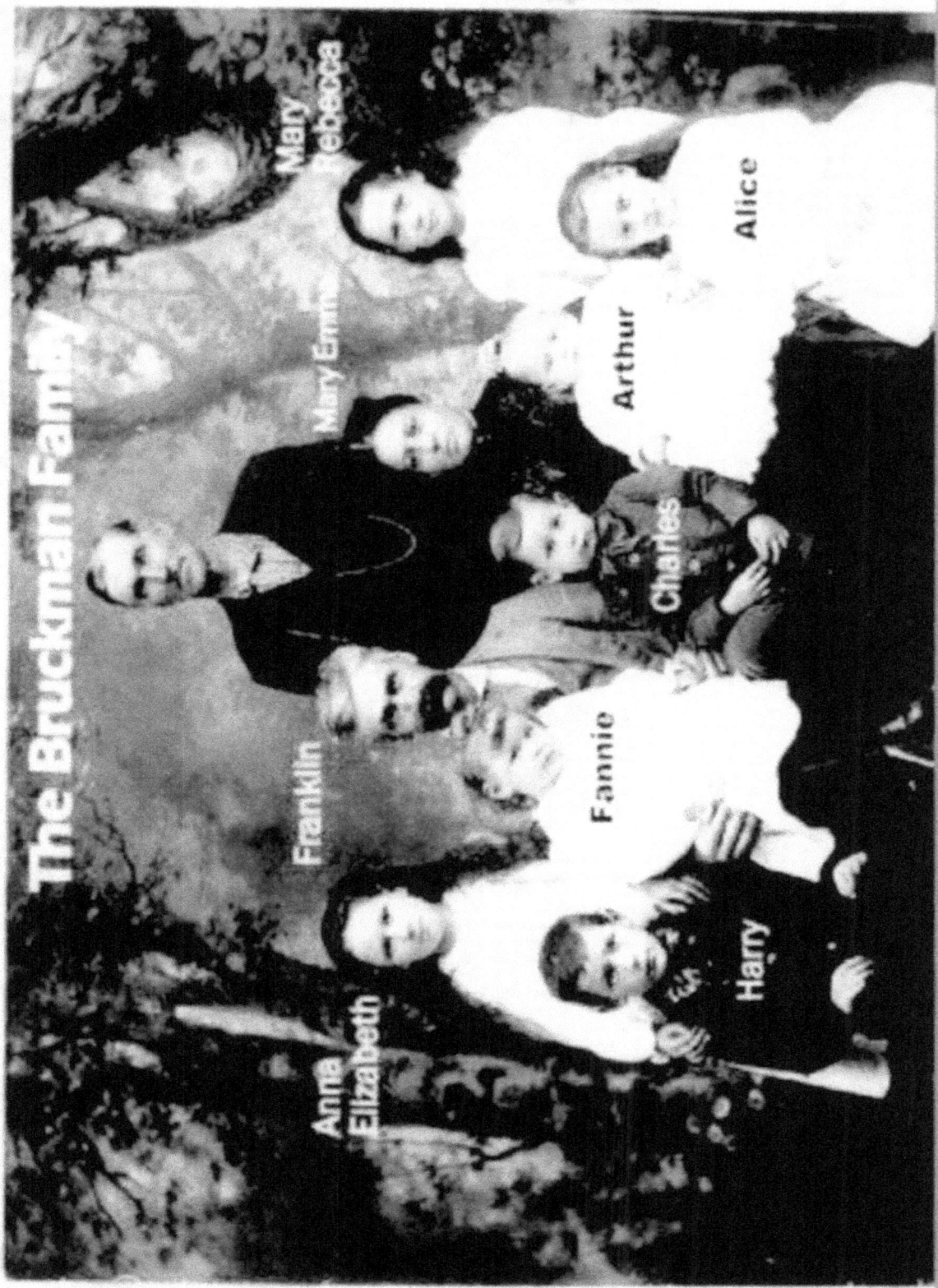

The Bruckman Family

Mary
Rebecca
Alice
Arthur
Mary Emma
Charles
Franklin
Fannie
Anna
Elizabeth
Harry

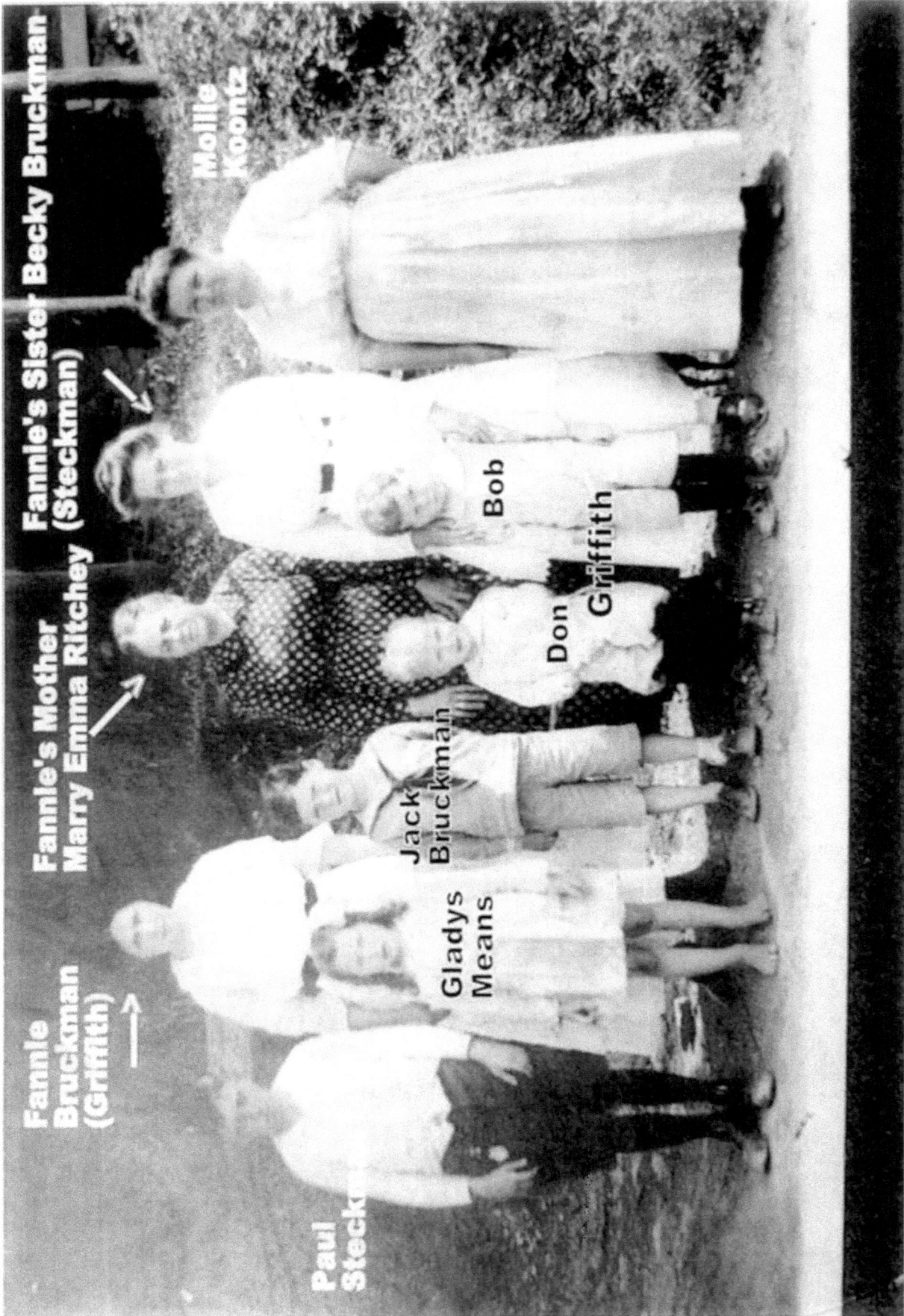

Fannie Bruckman (Griffith)

Fannie's Mother
Marry Emma Ritchey

Fannie's Sister Becky Bruckman (Steckman)

Mollie Koontz

Paul Steckman

Gladys Means

Jack Bruckman

Don

Bob

Griffith

48

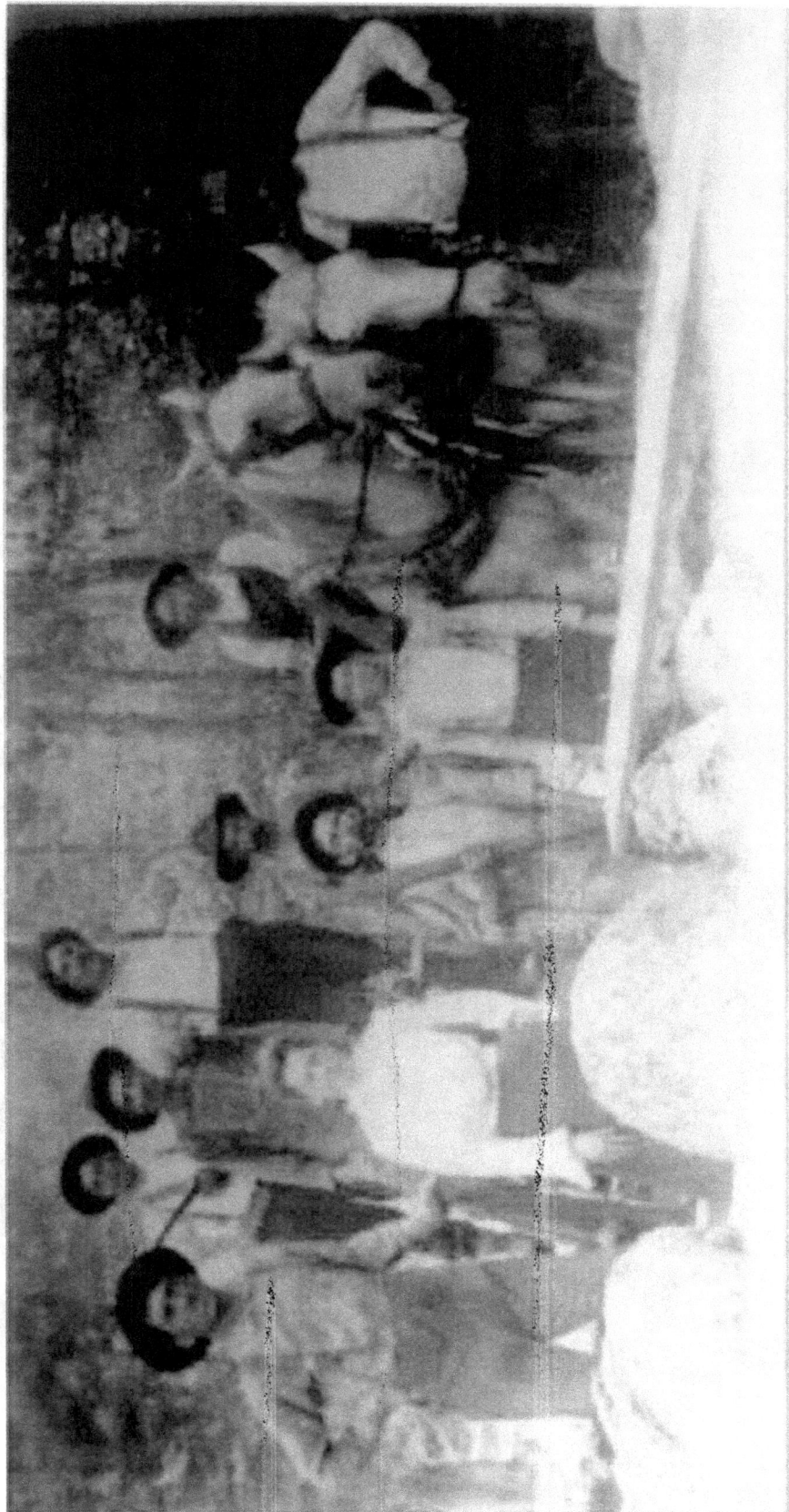

MARY EMMA (RITCHEY) BRUCKMAN and unknown others

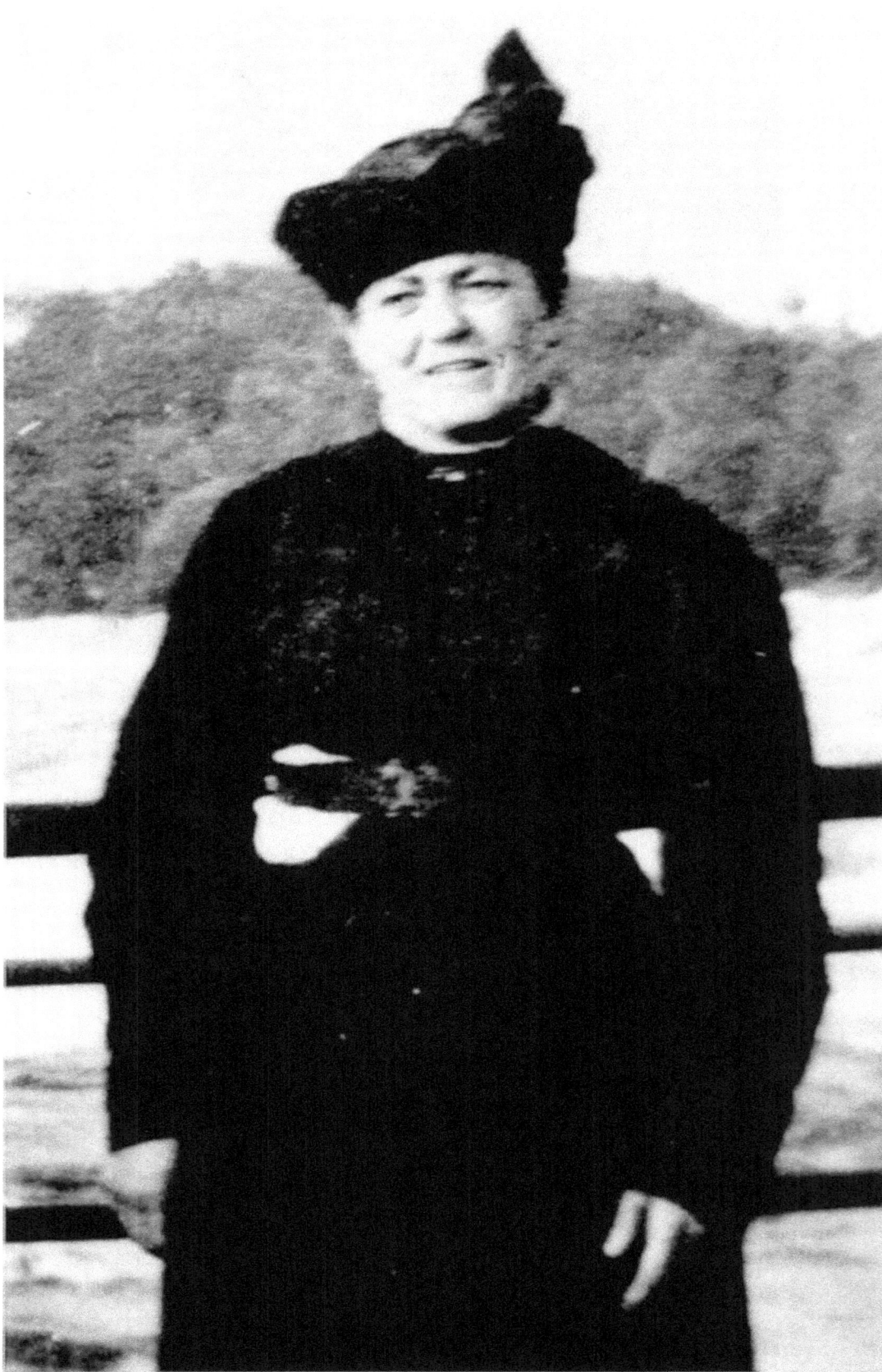

MARY EMMA (RITCHEY) BRUCKMAN

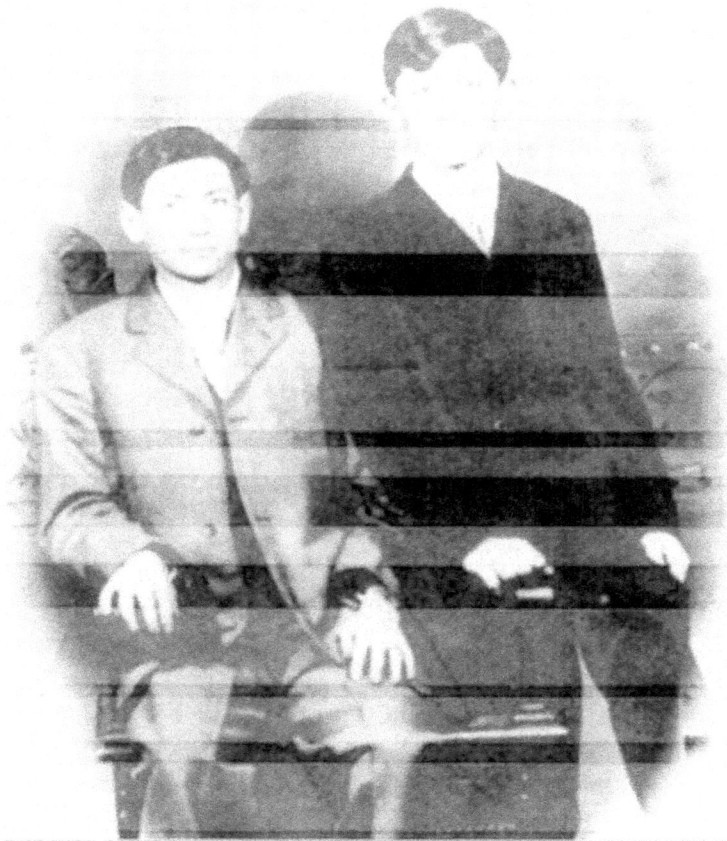

CHARLES HERBERT and ARTHUR FRANKLIN BRUCKMAN

Franklin D. Bruckman.

Franklin D. Bruckman, a well known school teacher, died at Harrisburg November 3, 1899, and was buried at Everett, his home, on Sunday last. The deceased was born in Salisbury, Somerset county, June 27, 1849 He was educated in the public schools of that town, and since he was eighteen years of age has been teaching school during the winter term. He was a carpenter by trade and followed that occupation during the summer. He was appointed storekeeper and gauger in 1884 and served four years. During this time he resided in Bedford. While teaching in Bean's Cove last winter his mind became deranged and he was sent to Harrisburg for treatment, but did not seem to improve. Mr. Bruckman was a brother of Mrs. Dr. A. Enfield, of Bedford. He is survived by a wife and several children.

The Bedford Gazette 10 Nov 1899

MRS. MARY EMMA BRUCKMAN

Mrs. Mary Emma Bruckman, widow of Franklin D. Bruckman, died at the Altoona hospital Monday night, death being caused by Bright's disease after a long illness. She was born near Everett, Bedford county, October 18, 1862, a daughter of Philip and Mary Ritchey, both deceased. Surviving are the following children: Mrs. C. H. Steckman, of this city; Mrs. J. A. Means, of Everett; Harry V. Bruckman, of Sproul; Mrs. Alice Beasom and Charles H., Arthur F. and John E. Bruckman, all of this city, and Mrs. R. R. Griffith, of Eldorado. Sixteen grandchildren and the following brothers and sisters also survive: Mrs. Elizabeth Kennard, of Clearville; Mrs. William Crawford and Mrs. John Ritchey, both of Everett; Mrs. Amanda Way, of Pitcairn; Samuel, William and Joseph Ritchey, of Everett. She attended the Gospel Hall of Altoona. Funeral services will be held at the home of her daughter, Mrs. C. H. Steckman, of 3124 Broad avenue, at 7.30 o'clock Wednesday evening. The remains may be viewed at the Steckman home until noon Thursday, when the body will be taken to Everett for interment. (Bedford county papers copy.)

Altoona Tribune 05 Sep 1923

51

MARTHA JANE BRUCKMAN was born on 09 Jul 1854, Salisbury, Somerset Co., PA and died 22 Sep 1919 in Salisbury, Somerset Co., PA. She married HOWARD WILLIAM DELOZIER on 16 May 1875, PA, son of TERRANCE DELOZIER and JULIA WEAKLAND. He was born on 28 May 1850 in Cambria Co., PA and died 06 Feb 1931 in Salisbury, Somerset Co., PA. Both are buried in Salisbury IOOF Cemetery, Salisbury, Somerset Co., PA.

Children of MARTHA BRUCKMAN and HOWARD DELOZIER are:

i. ROSE P. DELOZIER (E41)

ii. GEORGE GERBER DELOZIER (E42)

iii. LUCY MAY DELOZIER (E43)

iv. TORRENCE B. DELOZIER (E44) was born in Apr 1880 in Somerset Co., PA and died 22 May 1880 in Somerset Co., PA. Old Salisbury Cemetery, Salisbury, Somerset Co., PA.

v. VIRGIL HOMER. DELOZIER (E45) was born on 13 Jun 1882 in Somerset Co., PA and died 22 Sep 1933 in Greenville Twp., Somerset Co., PA. He was never married.

vi. FRANK HOWARD DELOZIER (E46) was born on 13 Mar 1883 in Somerset Co., PA and died 22 May 1928 in Somerset Twp., Somerset Co., PA. He was never married.

vii. WALTER A. DELOZIER (E47)

viii. ALICE R. DELOZIER (E48)

ix. ADA A. DELOZIER (E49)

x. FANNY GRACE DELOZIER (E4A) was born in Mar 1891in Somerset Co., PA and died in 1930 in ND.

xi. JULIA RUTH DELOZIER (E4B) was born in Apr 1893 in Somerset Co., PA and died in CO.

xii. HELEN BLANCHE DELOZIER (E4C) was born in 1894 in Somerset Co., PA.

Ref: 26, 7-Salisbury Somerset Co PA F54, 8-Elk Lick Twp (east part) Salisbury Somerset Co PA F9, 9-Salisbury Somerset Co PA F3, 27-D-HWD-18854, 27-D-MJB-96154, 27-D-VHD-82102, 27-D-FHD-55673, 44, 45, 46

Salisbury Loses Sterling Citizen
Howard DeLozier Passes Away Unexpectedly - Was Noted for His Joviality Was One of Youngest Veterans of Civil War Howard William DeLozier, who was a jovial and picturesque character in and about Salisbury for considerably more than a half-century, died shortly after 7 o'clock p.m., Feb. 6, 1931, at the age of 80 years, 8 months and 27 days. He was born May 28, 1850, in Carroll Township, Cambria County, Pa. He was a son of the late Terrance and Julia

Weakland DeLozier. Mr. DeLozier came to Salisbury in 1875. He was attracted here by the shook industry, with which he was identified for some years, both in the woods and in the shook shops, cutting the timber which was split into staves, and later shaped up in the shook shops for making casks to contain molasses and rum. The staves were all exported to Cuba, enough in each bundle, or shook, to make one cask. There was no more healthful labor than that which was associated with the shook industry. Owing to the fact that Mr. DeLozier during the years of his young manhood followed an exceptionally healthful occupation, and the additional fact that he was born with a strong, vigorous constitution, it was but natural that he possessed health and strength beyond that of the average person, and carried much of it with him almost to the brink of the grave. He was ill but little during his entire lifetime, and for that reason his death came as a great surprise, as his final illness set in only a few days before he closed his eyes upon earth's fitful scenes forever. Only four days before he died he was about town in his usual jovial mood. He seemed to have a cold, and expressed to some of his friends the opinion that he was getting grip or some similar malady, but did not seem to think it would develop into anything serious. However, a day or two later he took to his bed, and a day or two before he died seemed to become paralyzed in his throat and other parts of his body, and soon lapsed into coma. At no time after taking to his bed did he have much desire to talk, or seem to take much interest in anything or those about him. When he was averse to talking, joking or laughing, he was not only ill, but very ill. When the Civil War broke out, Howard DeLozier was only eleven years old, and when he was only a few weeks past his fourteenth year he was a stalwart "6-footer," and had no trouble in getting into the United States Army as a volunteer soldier, he and his father enlisting at the same time, in Co. C, 209th Infantry Regiment, wherein they served their country well, and were honorably discharged after serving the full time for which they had enlisted. Howard DeLozier was still a young man when he came to Salisbury in 1875 as a shook-maker, and worked in a shop operated here by the late William Smith. The same year he married Martha Bruckman, a daughter of the late Dr. and Mrs. J. G. Bruckman. To them twelve children were born. Mrs. DeLozier died in September, 1919. The following named children survive: Rose, wife of the late William Petry, of Johnstown; George G., of Glencoe; Lucy, wife of Arthur Sharp, Meyersdale; Virgil, who has no established residence; Walter, and Ada, wife of George Schrock, Johnstown; Grace, of North Dakota; Ruth, of Colorado. Four of their children, Terrence, Frank, Blanche and Mrs. Alice Mull preceded the parents in death. Several years after the death of his wife, Mr. DeLozier took unto himself a second wife in the person of Mrs. Ellen Harrison, who lived only about two or three years. After being a widower for another period of a few years, Mr. DeLozier married again, his third wife being Mrs. Mary Trent, who had also been married twice before becoming the wife of her third husband, whom she survives, with six sons, three of whom were fathered by her first husband, the late Alexander Facenbaker, and three by her second husband, the late Hesekiah Trent. Mrs. DeLozier is a daughter of the late Christian Bower, and some of her children are quite young, the youngest being only about five years old. The surviving wife of the deceased is many years younger than her third husband was, but she was very devoted to him, as he also was to her, and they lived very happily together during the three years and nearly five months which intervened between their marriage and the aged husband's death. Howard DeLozier was a remarkable man in many ways. Though a man of rough exterior, and almost brutally frank in expressing his opinions at times, he had many most excellent traits, and though rough and "hardboiled," so to speak, in some respects, there was a big, kind heart back of his rough exterior, and he was always ready to do a kind turn, or to help anyone in distress to the extent of his ability. Moreover, he was a useful citizen, as well as an honest one. From the time he was big enough to work, almost to his dying day, he was generally busy at something, and was able to turn his hand to almost anything, and was a strong worker at whatever he turned his hand to. After the shook industry came to an end in this locality, he worked to some extent among the farmers, also worked in the mines for a good many years, followed teaming to some extent, and also for a number of years served the farmers of this locality as a veterinary surgeon. As a veterinarian he acquired the title of "Doc," and was known to almost every man, woman and child in Salisbury and vicinity as "Doc DeLozier." He also served his fellow citizens of Salisbury as Burgess, and in various other official capacities at various times. He was not only a useful citizen, but a highly amusing one, as he possessed a large humorous streak in his make-up, lots of ready wit, and was the dispenser of much quaint and humorous philosophy. Truly, he was a picturesque character, very outspoken, at times very saracastic, sometimes quickly moved to anger, but just as quick to forgive an injury, and he never nursed a grudge. In addition to his surviving wife, children and step-children, Mr. DeLozier is also survived by about thirty grandchildren, about ten great-grandchildren and brothers and sisters as follows: James, of Greensburg; Ignatius, Raphael and Mrs. Julian Wortham of Altoona, and Mrs. Amelia Leene, of Pittsburgh. The funeral service was held at the DeLozier residence on Corliss Street, Sunday afternoon at 3:45 o'clock, conducted by Rev. S. D. Sigler of St. John's Lutheran Church. The burial arrangement was in charge of Funeral Director J. L. Tressler, of Meyersdale, assisted by the Sons of Veterans, who arranged for a military burial. That Howard William DeLozier had many friends, was plainly shown by the large number of persons in attendance at the funeral, many coming from other communities. Most of his children and other near relatives attended the funeral, but some found it impossible to be there.

Meyersdale Republican 12 Feb 1931

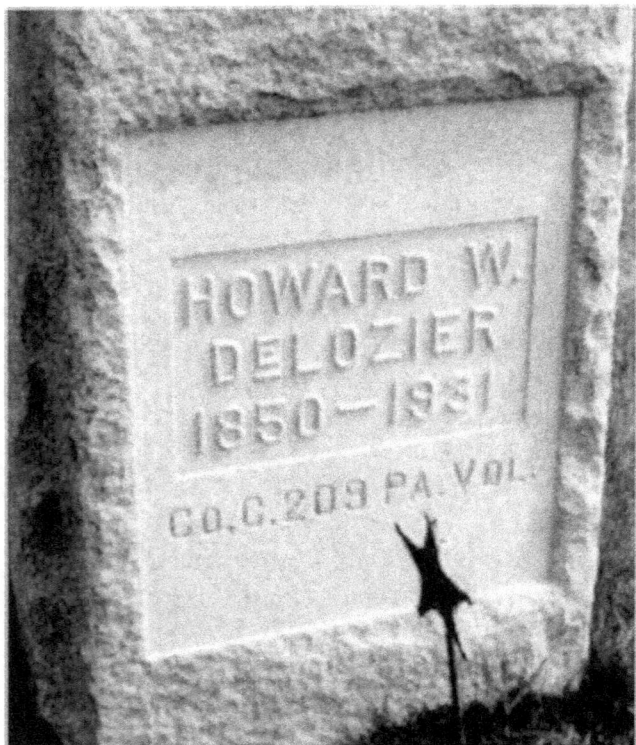

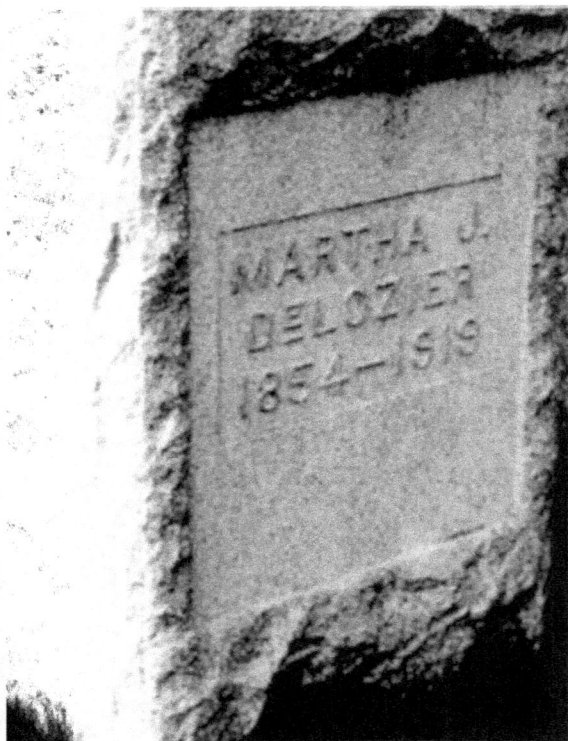

Delozier, Howard W.   (3-M-6)

Widow.

Minor.   *Delozier, Mary*   (Next friend)

C. 209 Pa. Inf

DATE OF FILING.	CLASS.	APPLICATION NO.	CERTIFICATE NO.	STATE FROM WHICH FILED.
1891 Mar 27	Invalid,	1010 173	976 319	Pa.
	Widow,			
1931 Jan 20	Minor.	1689.035		Pa.

Attorney: *J.B. Cralle Co.*

XC 2 639 862

Name: Howard W DeLozier; Residence: Pennsylvania; Enlistment Date: 8 Sep 1864; Rank at enlistment: Private; State Served: Pennsylvania; Survived the War?: Yes; Service Record: Enlisted in Company C, Pennsylvania 209th Infantry Regiment on 08 Sep 1864.Mustered out on 31 May 1865 at Alexandria, VA.; Sources: History of Pennsylvania Volunteers, 1861-1865

FORM MAGO 41 5M 12-380 Commonwealth of Pennsylvania Department of Military Affairs	RECORD OF BURIAL PLACE OF VETERAN	Somerset County

NAME DeLozier, Howard W	DATE OF BIRTH May 27, 1840	DATE OF DEATH Feb. 6, 1931

VETERAN OF   WAR   SERVED IN

Civil   ARMY (X) NAVY ( ) MARINE CORPS ( )

DATES OF SERVICE 9/8/64 5/31/65	ORGANIZATION (S) Co. C 209 Pa. Vol.	RANK Private

CEMETERY OR PLACE OF INTERMENT

NAME   I.O.O.F.

LOCATION   Salisbury Pa.

LOCATION OF GRAVE IN CEMETERY   HEADSTONE

SECTION LOT No. S.Center   RANGE GRAVE No.   GOVERNMENT ( ) COUNTY ( ) FAMILY (X)

INFORMATION GIVEN BY   Bates Hist.   REMARKS

DATE 12/4/34

After being Recorded in the County Veterans' Grave Registration Record This card is to be sent to THE ADJUTANT GENERAL'S OFFICE, Harrisburg, Pennsylvania, for final Record.

DeLozier   Howard

E21 WALTER F. ENFIELD E2

Dr. WALTER F. ENFIELD was born on 31 Mar 1872 in Somerset Co., PA and died 11 Apr 1941 Bedford, Bedford Co., PA. He married MARGARET IRWIN on 03 Jun 1896 in Bedford County, PA, daughter of JAMES M. IRWIN and MARY HAMILTON. She was born on 25 Jan 1870 in Huntingdon, Huntingdon Co., PA and died 30 Oct 1936 in Bedford, Bedford Co., PA. He left a will recorded in Book 18, Page 77, Bedford County Courthouse, Bedford, Bedford Co., PA

Children WALTER ENFIELD and MARGARET IRWIN are:

i. THOMAS W. ENFIELD (E211)

ii. GEORGE STEWART ENFIELD (E212)

iii. HELEN FRANCES ENFIELD (E213) was born in 1903 in Bedford, Bedford Co., PA.

iv. ROBERT FINLEY ENFIELD (E214)

Ref: 8-Ward West Bedford Bedford Co PA F29, 9-Ward West Bedford Bedford Co PA F102, 27-D-WFE-35850, 27-D-MMI-91701

MRS. ENFIELD DIES AT BEDFORD HOME
Funeral Services Held Sunday Afternoon At 2:00 O'clock
Funeral services were held Sunday afternoon at 2 o'clock at the Enfield home, South Richard street, for Mrs. Walter F. Enfield, who died Friday, October 30th, it 8:30 o'clock at her home after an illness of two months, death being attributed to a heart ailment. Her pastor, the Rev. Walter H. Williams of the Methodist church conducted the services, he was assisted by the Rev. Oscar F. R. Treder, rector of the, Episcopal church. Miss Emma, Shuck, a close friend of Mrs. Enfield sang, "Lead Kindly Light." The pall bearers were: Richard W. Lins, esq., A. S. Russell, Ira J. Powell, Victor E. P. Barkman, Shirley Hulse and Dr. Raymond Grissinger. Burial was made in Bedford cemetery. Mrs. Enfield's maiden name was Margaret Irwin; she was born in Huntingdon, January 25, 1870, a daughter of James M. and Mary Irwin. She was a graduate of the Huntingdon High School. She was married to Dr. Enfield at Cumberland, Md., on June 3, 1896. Surviving are the husband and these children: Dr. Thomas W. Enfield of Phila., Dr. Geo. S. Enfield of Bedford, Miss Helen Enfield and Robert Enfield, both of Bedford, and two grand children, Charlottee Enfield of Philadelphia and Stuart Enfield of Bedford. Mrs. Enfield was the last surviving member of her family. She was a member of the Methodist church and of the Bedford county Federation of Women. Mrs. Enfield led a busy life. As the wife of a physician and mother of four children, her chief interest was always her home. She will long be remembered here as a lovable friend and neighbor and a model Christian wife and mother.
The Bedford Gazette 1936

E23 CHARLES L. ENFIELD E2

CHARLES L. ENFIELD was born on 21 Jul 1880 in Bedford Co., PA and died 12 Feb 1940 in Pittsburgh, Allegheny Co., PA. He married ADELINE "ADDA" MILLER, daughter of GEORGE MILLER and SARAH CAMPBELL. She is born in 1888 in McKeesport, PA and died 14 Apr 1944 in Pittsburgh, Allegheny Co., PA.

Child of CHARLES ENFIELD and ADELINE MILLER is:

i. REBECCA ENFIELD (E231)

Ref: 27-D-CLE-22198, 11- Pittsburgh Allegheny Co PA F650, 27-D-AM-41885

Charles L. Enfield

Bedford, Pa., Feb. 15—Charles L. Enfield, 63, a native of Bedford, died of lobar pneumonia at noon Monday at his home at 3913 Nantasker street, Pittsburgh. Burial took place yesterday morning in Bedford Cemetery.

Mr. Enfield was born here in July, 1876, a son of the late Dr. and Mrs. Americus Enfield. He was married in 1902 to Miss Ada Miller, who survives with one daughter, Rebecca, wife of Dr. Charles McDermott of Pittsburgh.

Mr. Enfield was a brother of Dr. Walter E. Enfield, Miss Fannie Enfield and Miss Olive Enfield, all of Bedford, and Mrs. Mary Legg of Hollywood, Fla.

Mr. Enfield was educated in the Bedford schools and was a member of the Reformed Church. For a time he was engaged in the insurance business here. He became a member of the G. S. Meyer Insurance Agency in McKeesport and later was in the office of the Federal Housing Board at Pittsburgh.

Cumberland Evening Times 15 Feb 1940

E31 MARY REBECCA BRUCKMAN E3

MARY REBECCA BRUCKMAN was born 15 Mar 1881 in Everett, Bedford Co., PA, and died 18 Feb 1957 in Bedford Co., PA. She married CHARLES H. STECKMAN 15 Dec 1904 in Everett, Bedford Co., PA, son of ANDREW STECKMAN and ELIZABETH _____. He was born 1882 in Everett, Bedford Co., PA.

Child of MARY BRUCKMAN and CHARLES STECKMEN is:

i. PAUL M. STECKMAN (E311)

Ref: 9-Ward 2 Altoona Blair Co PA F231, 10-Logan Twp Blair Co PA F312

MARK ANNIVERSARY ON WEDDING DATE

Mr. and Mrs. Charles H. Steckman of 3124 Broad Avenue Married Twenty-five Years Ago Yesterday:

Mr. and Mrs. Charles H. Steckman of 3124 Broad avenue yesterday observed their silver wedding anniversary and during the day entertained a total of forty-nine relatives and friends, who called in honor of the occasion, as guests in their home.

That the guests did not come empty handed and with words alone is demonstrated forcibly by the many valuable and useful gifts, many of them in silver, received by the celebrating couple. In addition Mr. and Mrs. Steckman presented each other with handsome watches.

Charles H. Steckman and Miss Mary Rebecca Bruckman were united in marriage in the home of the bride's mother, Mrs. M. E. Bruckman in Everett, on Dec. 15, 1904, Rev. F. I. Sigmund, Baptist pastor, officiating. They first established their home in Everett but for the past twenty-years have resided in Altoona, first at Seventh avenue and Fourteenth street and for th past fourteen years at the present location.

Mr. Steckman is well known in the city as well as over the entire Pennsylvania Railroad system as the holder of the quoit championship. He holds the title at the present time and in the past nine years has held the title for seven of nine years. The two years in which the title passed to other hands Mr. Steckman did not compete and thus has never yet been defeated in the quoit title bouts. He is employed in the South Altoona spring shop.

Among the gifts presented to Mr. and Mrs. Steckman was a large turkey and the fowl aided in providing food for many of the visitors at the home. Those who called upon Mr. and Mrs. Steckman yesterday were: Mr. and Mrs. John A. Means and their son and daughter Gladys and John C., Mr. and Mrs. Roy Means and daughter Betty, Mr. and Mrs. Dan Sparks and daughter Mabel and son Melvin and Mr. and Mrs. Emmett Barnett and daughter Jean and sons James and Junior, all of Everett.

Mr. and Mrs. Foster Kerr and sons Jimmy and Johnny, Mr. and Mrs. Harry Mann and daughter Julia, Mr. and Mrs. Harvey Mann, and Mr. and Mrs. B. F. Mann, all of Clearfield; Mr. and Mrs. P. M. Steckman of Altoona, son and daughter-in-law of Mr. and Mrs. C. H. Steckman; Miss Fannie and Milton Enfield of Bedford; Mr. and Mrs. Walter Pennell of Johnstown; Mr. and Mrs. Boyd Coltabaugh and daughter Thelma and son Girard, of this city.

Mr. and Mrs. W. H. Russell, Mr. and Mrs. J. E. Miller, Mrs. Ed Brashears, Mr. and Mrs. A. Delozier and daughters Mary and Virginia, all of this city.

Altoona Mirror 16 Dec 1929

E32 ANNA ELIZABETH BRUCKMAN E3

ANNA ELIZABETH BRUCKMAN was born on 02 Mar 1882 in Everett, Bedford Co., PA and died 03 Mar 1972 in Everett, Bedford Co., PA. She married JOHN AMERICUS MEANS on 19 Apr 1905 in Bedford Co., PA. He was born on 05 May 1877 in Black Valley, PA and died 02 Nov 1949 in Everett, Bedford Co., PA. He is buried in Bethel Frame Church Cemetery, Clearville, Bedford Co., PA. He had a son ROY E. MEANS by his 1st wife NANCY STECKMAN.

Children of ANNA BRUCKMAN and JOHN MEANS are:

i. IVAN B. MEANS (E321)

ii. GLADYS R. MEANS (E322)

iii. JOHN C. MEANS (E323) was born 1922 in Monroe Twp., Bedford Co., PA.

Ref: 26, 8-Monroe Twp Bedford Co PA F46, 9-Monroe Twp Bedford Co PA F1, 10-Monroe Twp Bedford Co PA F167, 11-Monroe Twp Bedford Co PA F12

John A. Means

John American Means died Tuesday, Nov. 2 at his home in Black Valley.

He was born May 5, 1877, in Black Valley, a son of George and Anna (Koontz) Means He was first married to Nancy Steckman. After her death he was married to Elizabeth Bruckman April 19, 1905.

He is survived by his second wife and these children: Roy E. Means, Everett; Ivan B., Everett Star Rt.; John C., Pikesville, Md, and Mrs. Gladys Mills, Clearville Also surviving are three sisters: Mrs. Mary Grove and Mrs Lyda O'Neal, Clearville, and Mrs Minnie E. Marston, St. Louis, Mo Membership was held in the Lutheran church.

Funeral services will be conducted at 2 o'clock Saturday afternoon

Bedford Gazette 04 Nov 1949

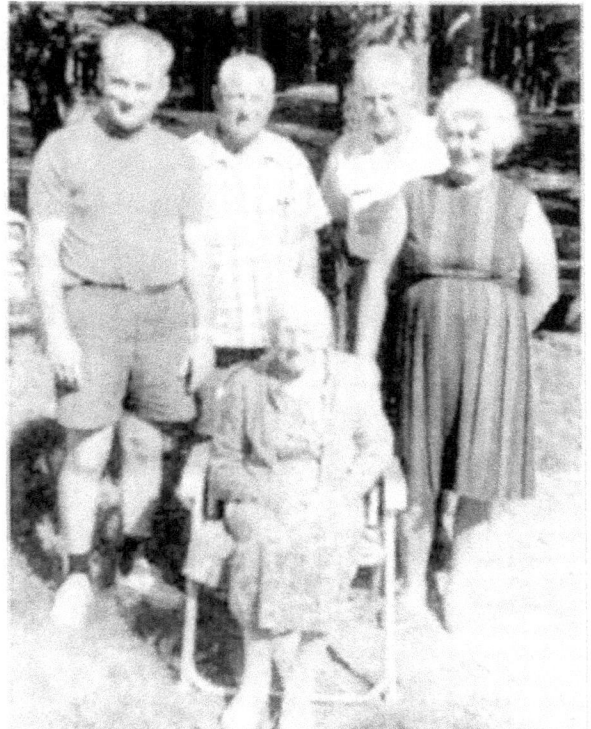

JOHN CHARLES MEANS, JOHN BRUCKMAN, IVAN MEANS & GLADYS R. (MEANS) MILLS and ANNA ELIZABETH (BRUCKMAN) MEANS

E33 HARRY VINCENT BRUCKMAN E3

HARRY VINCENT BRUCKMAN was born 23 Oct 1883 in Clearville, Bedford Co., PA, and died 09 Jan 1959 in Sproul, Blair Co., PA. He married DAISY MOSS MOORE, daughter of WILLIAM SAMUEL MOORE and ANNIE MOSS, on 25 Dec 1913 in Deseronto, Lennox, Ontario, Canada. She was born 1890 in Canada, and died 1948 in Sproul, Blair Co., PA.

Children of HARRY BRUCKMAN and DAISY MOORE are:

i. GRANT BRUCKMAN (E331)

ii. LOIS BRUCKMAN (E332)

Ref: 10-Greenfield Twp Blair Co PA F59, 11-Greenfield Twp Blair Co PA F67

FORM 2.

AFFIDAVIT.

(I George V., Cap. 52.)

Required before License or Certificate is Granted by Issuer of Marriage Licenses by provision of

The Marriage Act.

005900

3. Harry Vincent Buckman of Altoona ... Blair, Pennsylvania, US ... spoke oath and say as follows:

1. I and Daisy Mura Moore ... Town of Deseronto ... of Hastings, Ontario ... are desirous of entering into a Contract of Marriage, and of having our Marriage duly solemnized at the Town of Deseronto ... of Hastings Ontario ...

2. According to the best of my knowledge and belief, there is no affinity, consanguinity, prior marriage or any other lawful cause or legal impediment to bar or hinder the solemnization of the said Marriage.

3. Daisy Mura Moore ... is of the municipality of ... in the said County or District of Deseronto ... of Hastings

4. I am of the age of 30 years, and the said Daisy Mura Moore is of the full age of 18 years.

5. I am a Bachelor ... and the said Daisy Mura Moore is a Spinster ...

Sworn before me at Deseronto in the County of Hastings this 23rd day of November 1913

Bert M. Bruce, Issuer of Marriage Licenses at Deseronto

Harry Vincent Buckman

PARTICULARS TO BE SUPPLIED BY MINISTER, ETC.

BRIDEGROOM

Name	Harry Vincent Buckman
Age	30
Residence when Married	Altoona, Pa. U.S.A.
Place of Birth	United States, America
Bachelor or Widower	S
Occupation	Bricklayer
Religious Denomination	Brethren
Name of Father	Frank W. Buckman
Maiden Name of Mother	Emma M. Ritchey

BRIDE

Name	Daisy Mura Moore
Age	26
Residence when Married	Deseronto, Ont.
Place of Birth	Hastings
Spinster or Widow	S
Religious Denomination	Brethren
Name of Father	Wm. Sam. Moore
Maiden Name of Mother	Annie Moss
Signature of Bridegroom	Harry V. Buckman
Signature of Bride	Daisy G. Moore
Name of Witness	Mrs. Wilbur Moore
Address	Deseronto
Name of Witness	Wilbur M. Moore
Address	Deseronto

I certify the above named parties were married by me at Deseronto in the county of Hastings this 25th day of Nov. 1913

Signature Robert Burns

Address Box 372 Deseronto Ont.

Denomination Methodist

60

FATHER
HARRY V. BRUCKMAN
1883 — 1959
JESUS SAVES

MOTHER
DAISY M BRUCKMAN
1889 — 1948
CHRIST DIED FOR THE UNGODLY

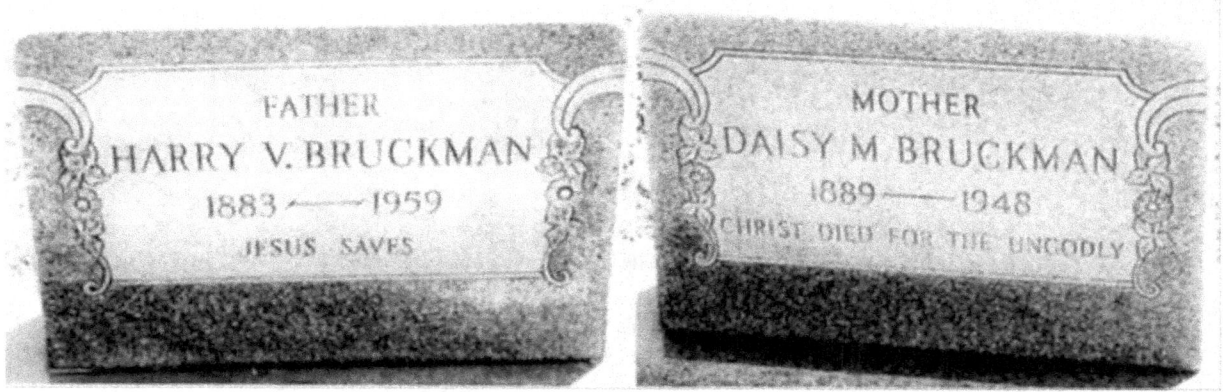

E34 ALICE MAY BRUCKMAN E3

ALICE MAY BRUCKMAN was born 07 Jan 1885 in Everett, Bedford Co., PA, and died 08 May 1949 in Altoona, Blair Co., PA. She is buried in Carson Valley Cemetery, Duncansville, Blair Co., PA. She married (1) KENNETH BISHOP BEASOM, on 21 Apr 1915 in Altoona, Blair Co., PA, son of HERMAN BEASOM and CLARA _____. He was born 22 Aug 1887 in PA and died in 25 Nov 1922 in Altoona, Blair Co., PA. He is buried in Fairview Cemetery, Altoona, Blair Co., PA. She married (2) BOYD E. COLTABOUGH. She was a saleswoman in a department store.

Children of ALICE BRUCKMAN and KENNETH BEASOM are:

i. THELMA A. BEASOM (E341) was born in Jul 1917 in Blair Co., PA. She married JOHN RHODES. He was born in 1914 in PA.

ii. KENNETH GIRARD BEASOM (E342)

Ref: 26, 27-D-KBB-161735, 10-Logan Twp Blair Co PA F27, 11-Altoona Blair Co PA F93, 12-Ward 4 Altoona Blair Co PA F386

RECENT WEDDINGS

Beasom—Bruckman.
Mr. Kenneth Bishop Beasom, of this city and employed by the Baker estates, and Miss Alice May Bruckman, of 823 Second avenue, were married Wednesday evening at 9:30 o'clock at the home of the bride's parents by the Rev. W. S. Long, of the Sixth Avenue Brethren church. A number of friends witnessed the ceremony and an excellent dinner followed. Following a trip to eastern cities the newlyweds will return and reside in their new home at Rosclawn.

Altoona Tribune 23 Apr 1915

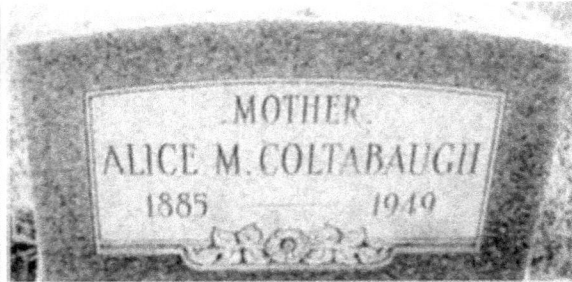

MRS. ALICE COLTABOUGH

Of 915 Seventh avenue, died in the Altoona hospital at 3.15 o'clock yesterday morning. Mrs. Coltabough was born in Bedford Jan. 7, 1885, the daughter of Franklyn and Emma (Richie) Bruckman. Her first husband, Kenneth Benson, preceded her in death a number of years ago. Surviving are her second husband, Boyd Coltabough; one son, Kenneth B. Benson of Altoona; a daughter, Mrs. Thelma A. Rhodes of Hollidaysburg; four grandchildren, three sisters, Mrs. John A. Means of Everett, Pa.; Mrs. R. R. Griffin and Mrs. C. H. Steckman, both of Altoona, and four brothers, H. B. Bruckman of Sproul, J. E. of Baltimore, A. F. and C. H. Bruckman, both of Altoona. Frineds will be received at the Gilden-Barton funeral home after 7 o'clock this evening.

Altoona Mirror 09 May 1949

E35 CHARLES HERBERT BRUCKMAN E3

CHARLES HERBERT BRUCKMAN was born 21 Aug 1887 in Everett, Bedford Co., PA, and died 27 Feb 1971 in Hollidaysburg, Blair Co., PA. He married MARY IRENE DETWILER 20 May 1916 in Altoona, Blair Co., PA, daughter of HENRY DILLING DETWILER and ANNA MARY KYLE. She was born 24 Apr 1894 in Martinsburg, Blair Co., PA, and died 07 Mar 1971 in Altoona, Blair Co., PA. They are buried at Alto-Reste Park Cemetery. In 1930, they were residing at 1124 - 19th Avenue, Altoona, Blair Co., PA and later purchased as house at 1423 Washington Avenue, Altoona, Blair Co., PA. On 05 Jun 1917, he was working as Pennsylvania Railroad Clerk at Altoona, Blair Co., PA and on 01 Sep 1920, Appointed U.S. Mail Carrier at Altoona, Blair Co., PA. They were members of the First Church of the Brethren, Altoona, Blair Co., PA.

Children of CHARLES BRUCKMAN and MARY DETWILER are:

i. DANIEL ALBERT BRUCKMAN (E351)

ii. HAROLD HERBERT BRUCKMAN (E352) b. 25 Dec 1918, Altoona, Blair Co., PA; d. 14 Jun 1980, Miami, Dade Co., FL; m. HELEN ORR, 1953, Dade Co., FL; b. 28 Nov 1923, Shelbyville, Shelby Co., KY; d. 19 Apr 1953, Miami, Dade Co., FL. He was cremated and his ashes spread in the Atlantic Ocean near Miami, FL. She was a Reservations Agent for National Air Lines. No known descendants.

iii. PAUL RAYMOND BRUCKMAN (E353)

iv. PHYLLIS JEAN BRUCKMAN (E354) was born on 03 Jun 1927 in Altoona, Blair Co., PA and died 12 Nov 1935 in Altoona, Blair Co., PA. She is buried at Alto-Reste Park Cemetery, Altoona, Blair Co., PA.

v. DORIS FAYE BRUCKMAN (E355)

vi. PHILIP EUGENE BRUCKMAN (E356) b. 22 Jan 1933, Altoona, Blair Co., PA; d. 23 Jul 2002, Copley, Lehigh Co., PA; m. MARCELLA LILLIAN BAILEY, 02 Sep 1972, PA; b. 01 Jul 1934, Towanda, PA. He served between Jan 1950 - May 1955, USNR Jan 1950-May 1951 & USN May 1951-May 1955 and last served aboard the ship USS Currituck (AV-7), a seaplane tender. He retired for Western Electric Plant, Allentown, PA. He resided at 75 Magna Drive, Coplay, PA 18037. No known descendants.

Ref: 10-Allegheny Twp Blair Co PA, 10-La Vale Allegheny Co MD, 11-1st Ward Altoona Blair Co PA, 14, 16

Bruckman—Detwiler.
Mr. Charles H. Bruckman, of 823 Second avenue, and Miss Mary J. Detwiler, daughter of Mr. and Mrs. H. D. Detwiler, of Clover Creek, were united in marriage at noon Saturday at the Sixth avenue Church of the Brethren parsonage. The groom is employed by the Pennsy and his bride is an attractive and popular young woman. They will be at home to numerous friends at 3126 Broad avenue.

Altoona Tribune 22 May 1916

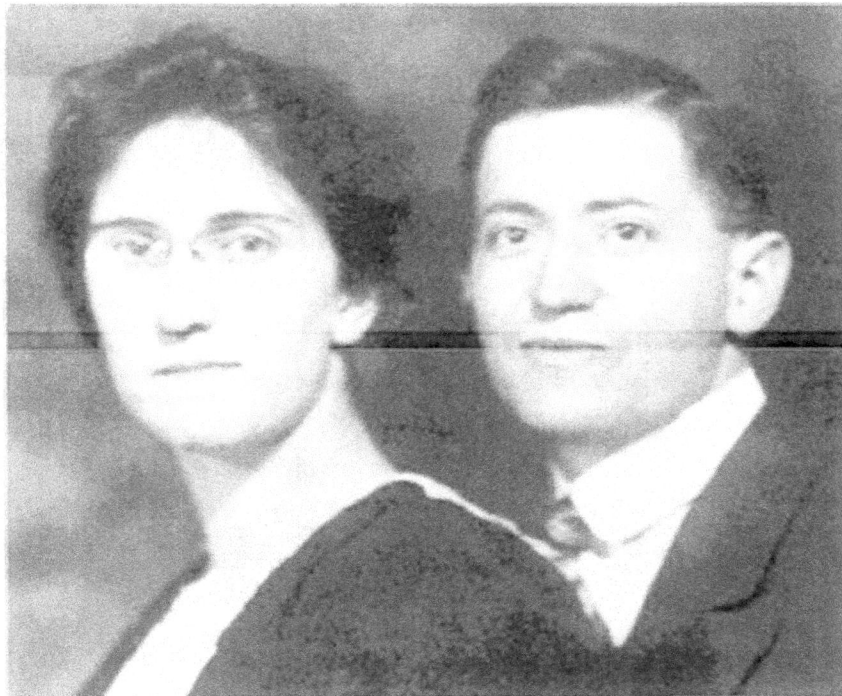

CHARLES HERBERT and MARY IRENE (DETWILER) BRUCKMAN

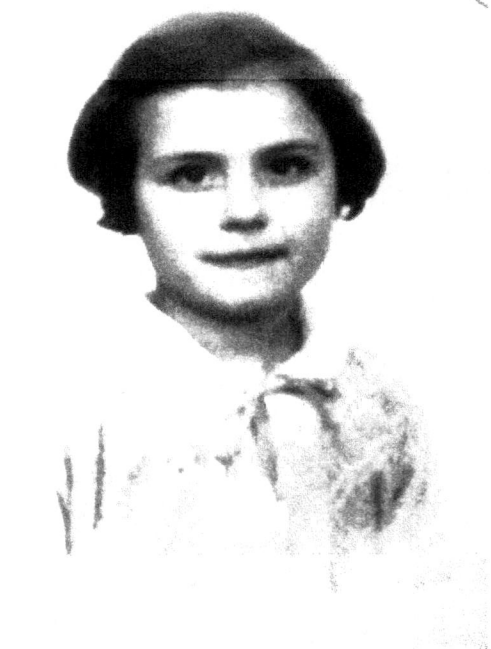

PHYLLIS JEAN BRUCKMAN

PHYLLIS JEAN BRUCKMAN

Phyllis Jean Bruckman, daughter of Charles H. and Mary (Detwiler) Bruckman, of 1124 Nineteenth avenue, died yesterday afternoon at 2:10 o'clock at the home, after a brief illness.

She was born in this city, June 3, 1927, and attended the Wright grade school and First Church of the Brethren Sunday school.

In addition to her parents, she is survived by the following brothers and sisters: Daniel, Harold Paul, Doris and Philip.

Funeral service will be held tomorrow afternoon at 2:30 o'clock at the home. The Rev. W. S. Long will officiate. Burial will be in Alto Reste Burial park.

Altoona Tribune 13 Nov 1935

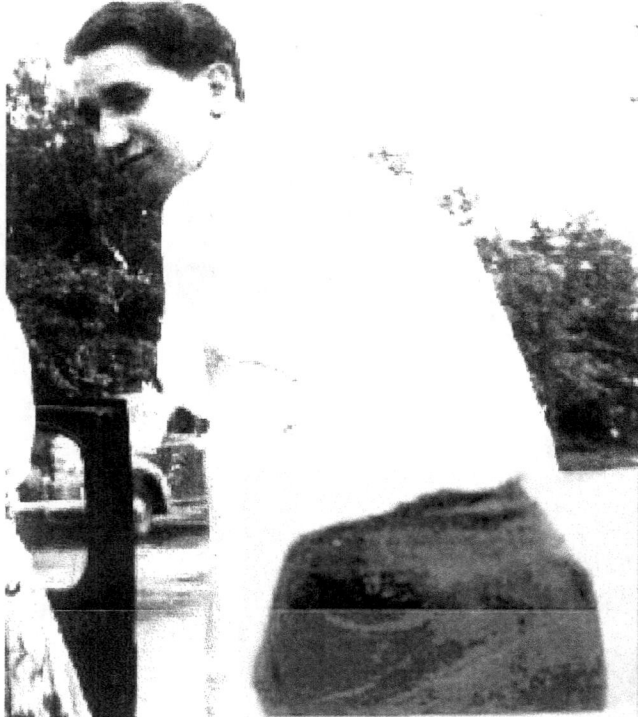

HAROLD HERBERT BRUCKMAN

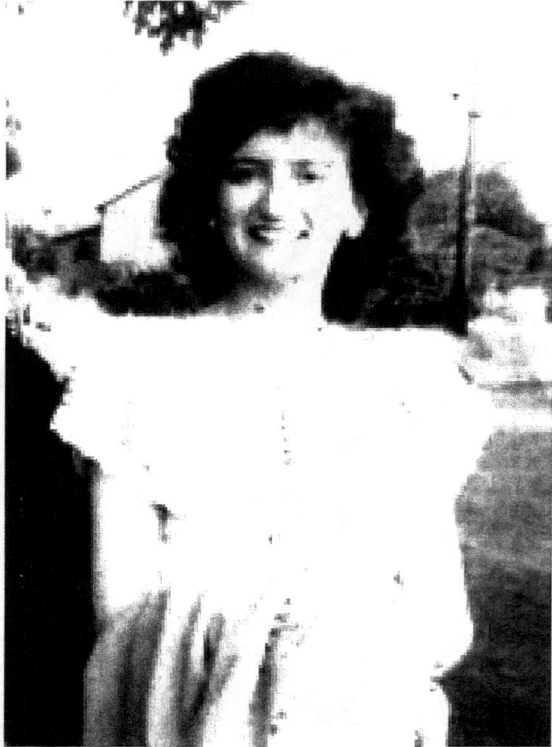

DORIS FAYE BRUCKMAN

64

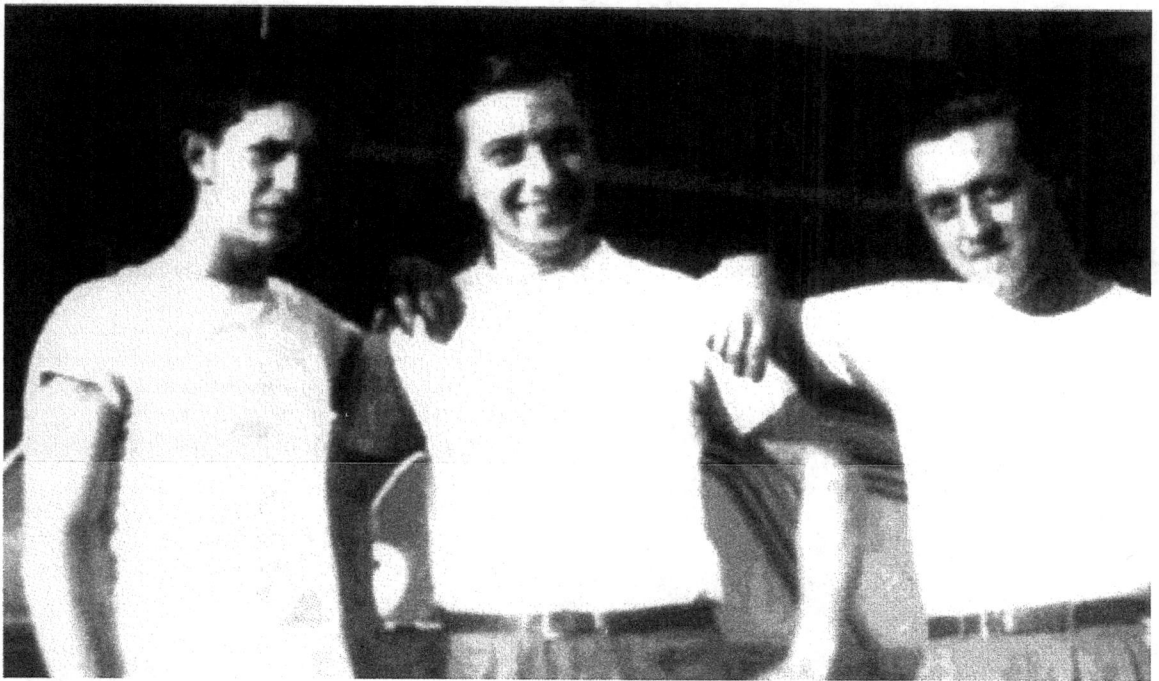

PHILIP EUGENE BRUCKMAN, DANIEL ALBERT BRUCKMAN and PAUL RAYMOND BRUCKMAN

Admiral Commends Altoona Sailor For Plane Crash Rescue

Philip E. Bruckman, seaman apprentice, USN, son of Mr. and Mrs. Charles Bruckman, 1423 Washington Ave., has been commended by the admiral in charge of his task force for rescuing two survivors from a burning seaplane that crashed into Guantanamo bay, Cuba.

Rear Adm. Richard F. Whitehead, USN, who commands the squadrons of long range patrol bombers tended by Bruckman's ship, the USS Currituck, said Bruckman "unhesitatingly and without further orders" took his boat to the crash scene although the aircraft was on fire and in danger of exploding.

The seaplane was a 32-ton twin engined Martin Mariner used in anti-submarine warfare. The remainder of the airmen were rescued by other Currituck boats.

The commendation follows:

"It has come to the attention of Commander-Fleet Air Wings, At-

(Continued on Page 4, Col. 7)

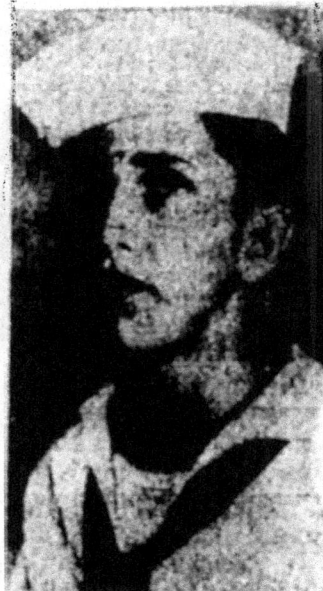

PHILIP E. BRUCKMAN

Admiral Commends Local Bluejacket

(Continued from Page 1)

lantic Fleet, that Bruckman, R. E., SA, USN, 3330238, was assigned as a member of the boat crew of the U. S. S. Currituck captain's gig on the morning of 1 February 1952, when a PBM seaplane of Utility Squadron Ten crashed into Guantanamo bay, Cuba.

"Records show that Bruckman's boat went immediately to the rescue, although the aircraft was burning and in danger of exploding. This action resulted in two survivors being rescued and later delivered ashore for medical attention.

"Commander Fleet Air Wings, Atlantic Fleet, wishes to commend Bruckman for the high order of seamanship, courage and devotion to duty, displayed by him as a crew member of the Currituck captain's gig, in the rescue operation described above.

"It is directed that this commendation be published at quarters, and be made a permanent part of subject man's service record."

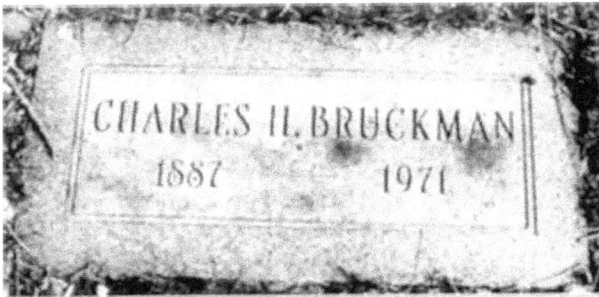

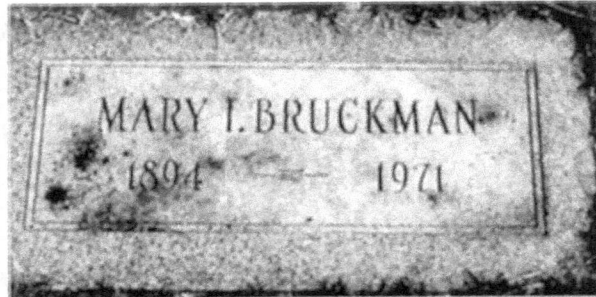

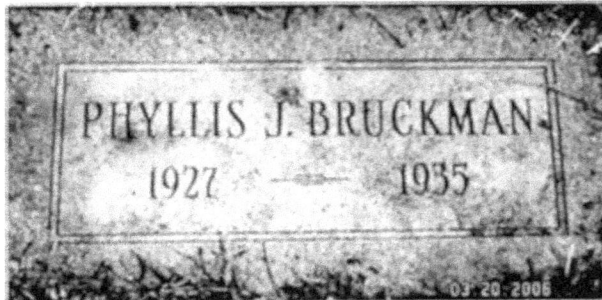

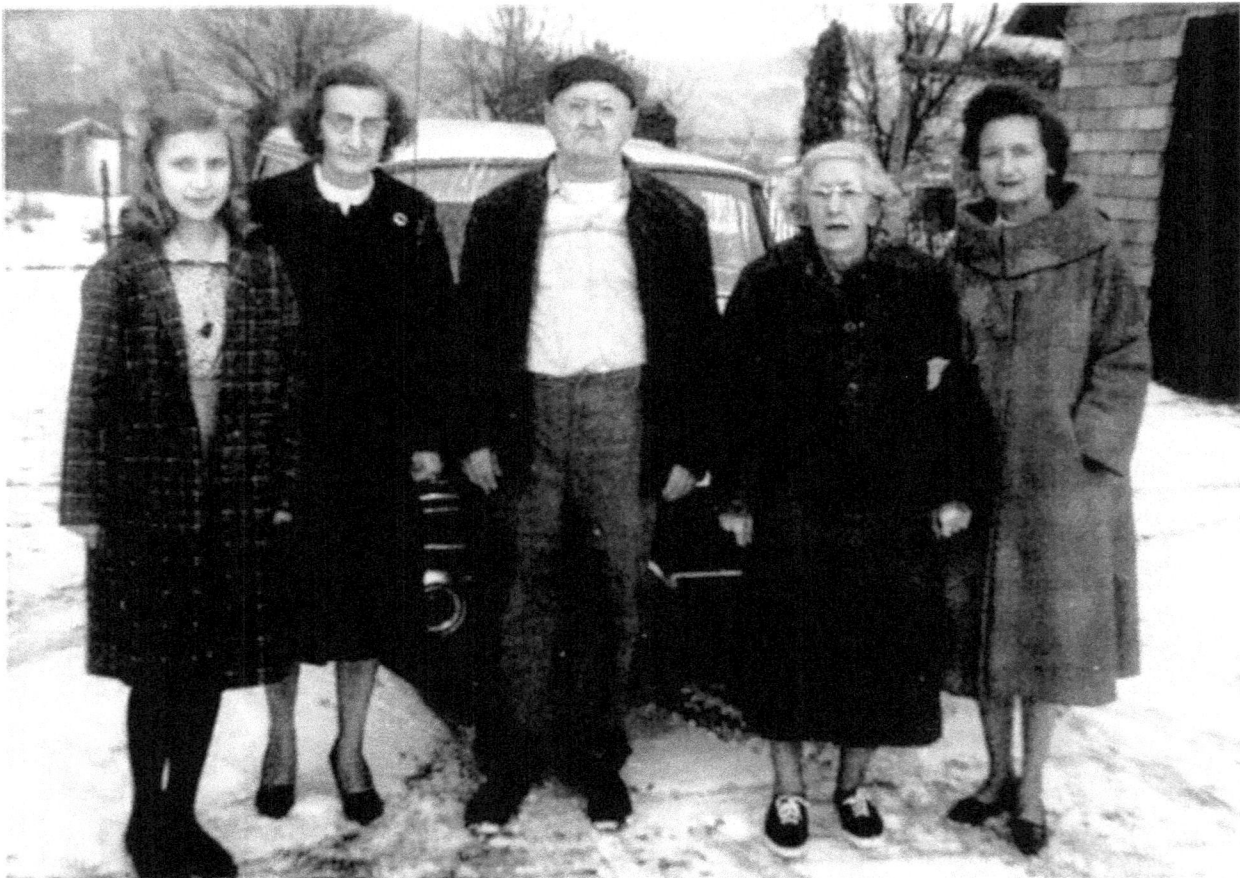

ESTHER MAY BRUCKMAN, JOSEPHINE LOUISE (BROWN) BRUCKMAN, CHARLES
HERBERT BRUCKMAN, MARY IRENE DETWILER and
DORIS "DORIE" (BRUCKMAN) LANTZ

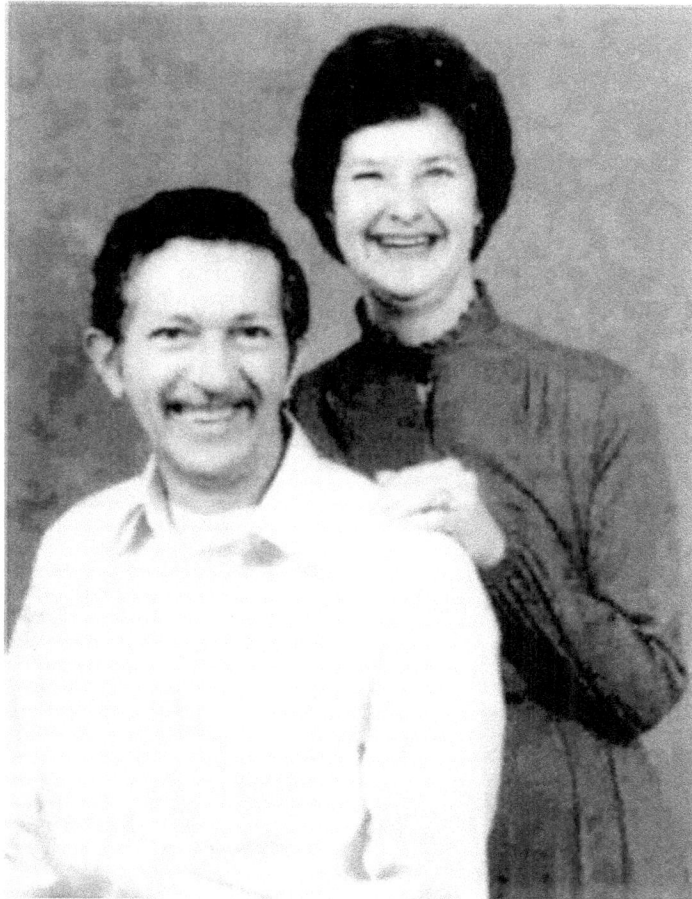

PHILIP EUGENE BRUCKMAN and
MARCELLA LILLIAN (BAILEY) BRUCKMAN

E36 FANNIE ZELUMA BRUCKMAN E3

FANNIE ZELUMA BRUCKMAN was born on 11 Mar 1889 in Everett, Bedford Co.,
PA and died on 12 May 1969 in Seattle, King Co., WA. She married RALPH RAYMOND
GRIFFITH, son of JOHN CALVIN GRIFFITH and EMMA LAVINA MOORE, on 01 Jul 1911
in Altoona, Blair Co., PA. He was born on 30 Jan 1887 in Fossilville, Bedford Co., PA and died
in 18 Mar 1959 in Seattle, King Co., WA.

Children of FANNIE BRUCKMAN and RALPH GRIFFITH are:

   i. ROBERT RALPH GRIFFITH (E361)

   ii. DONALD RICHARD GRIFFITH (E362)

   iii. ARTHUR RAYMOND GRIFFITH (E363)

Ref: 23-William Richard Griffith, 10-Logan Twp Blair Co PA F372, 11-Altoona Blair Co PA
F261, 12-Ward 14 Altoona Blair Co PA F304, 51

Altoona_Tribune 01 Jul 1911

Altoona Mirror 21 May 1969
(Note: Date of marriage incorrect.)

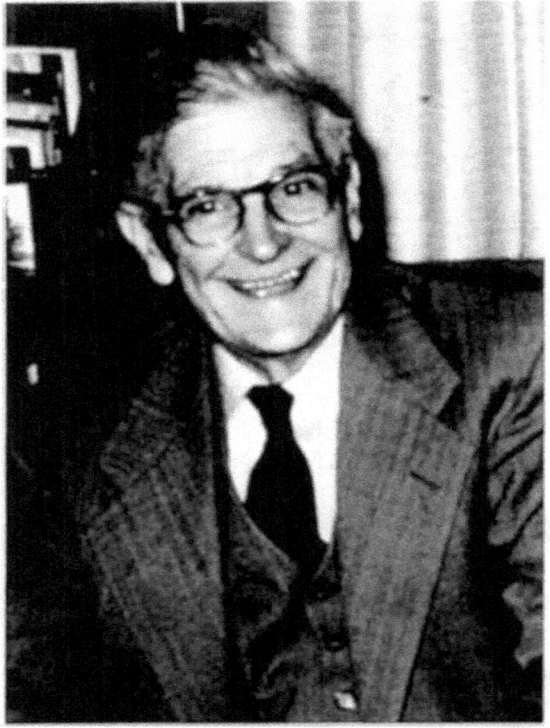

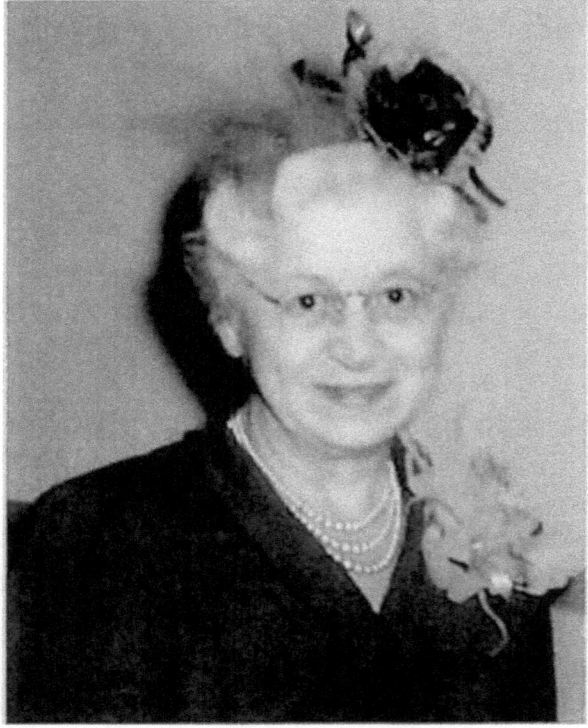

RALPH RAYMOND and FANNIE ZELUMA (BRUCKMAN) GRIFFITH

E37 ARTHUR FRANKLIN BRUCKMAN E3

ARTHUR FRANKLIN BRUCKMAN was born on 07 Dec 1891 in Everett, Bedford Co., PA and died 21 Feb 1950 in Altoona, Blair Co., PA. He married CAROLYN I. SWARTZ. She was born in 1893, PA and died in 1987 in PA. Both are buried at Alto-Reste Park Cemetery. She worked as a saleswoman in a department store in Altoona, Blair Co., PA.

Child of ARTHUR BRUCKMAN and CAROLYN SWARTZ is:

i. JACK RICHARD BRUCKMAN (E371)

Ref: 26

A. F. Bruckman

Arthur Franklin Bruckman, aged 58, well known proprietor of the Bruckman super-market in Altoona died unexpectedly at 12:45 o'clock Tuesday morning of a heart attack.

Mr. Bruckman was born in Bedford Dec. 7, 1891, a son of Frank D. and Emma (Ritchey) Bruckman but had spent almost all of his life in Altoona. He entered the service of the William F. Gable company as a cash boy and remained in the store employ for a period of 16 years.

Subsequently he established his own grocery store in the Eldorado area, the establishment growing into the modern super-market. He had been engaged in the grocery business for the past 25 years.

Surviving are his wife, Mrs. Carolyn (Swartz) Bruckman; a son, Jack, who was associated with his father in the operation of the market; two grandchildren, Thomas and Beverly, and the following brothers and sisters: Mrs. C. H. Steckman, Altoona; Mrs J. A. Means, of Everett; H. C. Bruckman, of Sproul; J. E. Bruckman, of Baltimore, Md.; Mrs. R. R. Griffith and C. H. Bruckman, of Altoona. A sister, Mrs Alice Coltabaugh, preceded him in death recently

Bedford Gazette 24 Feb 1950

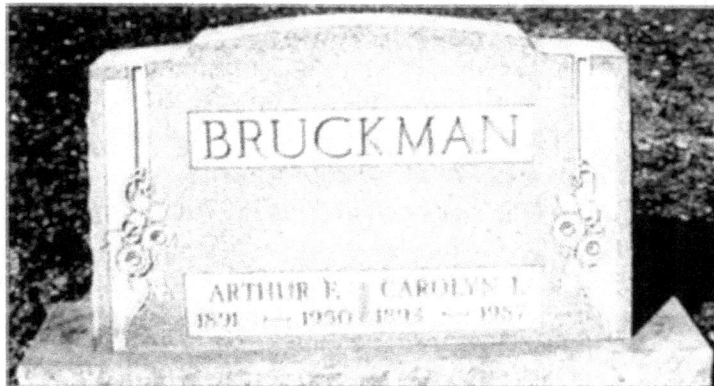

E38 JOHN ELLIS BRUCKMAN E3

JOHN ELLIS BRUCKMAN was born on 11 Mar 1894 in Everett, Bedford Co., PA and died Jan 1969 in Glen Bernie, Anne Arundel Co., MD. He married EDNA HELEN LAMCA, daughter of JOHN WILLIAM LAMCA and SARAH ELLEN MATTHEWS. She was born on 07 Aug 1896 in Altoona, Blair Co., PA and died 1955 in Glen Bernie, Anne Arundel Co., MD. He owned a butcher shop and was a salesman.

Children of JOHN BRUCKMAN and EDNA LAMCA are:

   i. RICHARD W. BRUCKMAN (E381)

   ii. ELOISE CLARECE BRUCKMAN (E382)

   iii. ROSELMA BRUCKMAN (E383)

Ref: 11-Altoona Blair Co PA F63, 12-Anne Arundel Co MD F362

MRS. EDNA LAMCA BRUCKMAN

Of 107 Main Ave., SW, Glen Burnie, Md., died Friday, May 6, after an extended illness. She was born in Altoona, Aug. 7, 1896, a daughter of the late John and Sarah Ellen (Matthews) Lamca.

She leaves her husband, John Bruckman; one son, Richard of Worthington, Md.; two daughters, Mrs. Eloise Kellenberger and Mrs. Roselma Felty, both of Glen Burnie; five grandchildren; three sisters, Mrs. Catherine Criste, Mrs. Ida Ferguson and Mrs. Grace Hays, all of Altoona. Two brothers, George and William Lamca and two sisters, Miss Mary Lamca and Mrs. Emma Tremmel, preceded her in death.

The funeral took place Tuesday at the Glen Burnie Methodist church.

Altoona Tribune 12 May 1955

E41 ROSE P. DELOZIER E4

ROSE P. DELOZIER was born on 28 Jan 1878 Somerset Co., PA and died 23 Jul 1936 in Johnstown, Cambria Co., PA. She married WILLIAM P. PETRY. He was born on 21 Jun 1867 in Germany and died 21 Oct 1929 in Johnstown, Cambria Co., PA.

i. ANNIE R. PETRY (E411) was born in Mar 1895 in Somerset Co., PA.

ii. GEORGE WILLIAM PETRY Sr. (E412)

iii. CHARLES R. PETRY (E413) was born in Aug 1897 in Somerset Co., PA.

iv. FLORENCE MAZIE PETRY (E414) was born on 23 Apr 1899 in Somerset Co., PA and died 25 Jan 1923 in Johnstown, Cambria Co., PA. She married CLOYD WIRICK. He was born in 1896 in PA. No children by this marriage.

v. MILDRED M. PETRY (E415) was born in 1912 in PA.

vi. HORACE H. PETRY (E416) was born on 24 Mar 1913 in PA and died 28 Jun 1976 in PA. He married LILLIAN _____. She was born 1916 in PA. He is buried in Forest Lawn Memorial Park, Johnstown, Cambria Co., PA.

U.S. World War II Army Enlistment Records, 1938-1946
Name: Horace H Petry
Birth Year: 1913
Race: White, citizen (White)
Nativity State or Country: Pennsylvania
State of Residence: Pennsylvania
County or City: Cambria
Enlistment Date: 13 Jul 1943
Enlistment State: Pennsylvania
Enlistment City: Altoona
Branch: No branch assignment
Branch Code: No branch assignment

Grade: Private
Grade Code: Private
Term of Enlistment: Enlistment for the duration of the War or other emergency, plus six months, subject to the discretion of the President or otherwise according to law
Component: Selectees (Enlisted Men)
Source: Civil Life
Education: 4 years of high school
Civil Occupation: Semiskilled chauffeurs and drivers, bus, taxi, truck, and tractor
Marital Status: Married
Height: 00
Weight: 000

Ref: 27-RPD-67655, 27-D-WPP-99867, 8-Paint Twp Somerset Co PA F178, 9-Ward 7 Johnstown Cambria Co PA F70, 10-Paint Twp Somerset Co PA F93, 27-D-FMP-8297, 10-Paint Somerset Co PA F94, 48

E42 GEORGE GERBER DELOZIER E4

GEORGE GERBER DELOZIER was born on 19 May 1877 in Salisbury, Somerset Co., PA and died 30 May 1946 in Glencoe, Somerset Co., PA. He married EMMA F. C. PETRY, daughter of FRANK F. PETRY and MARY WALKER. She was born on 21 Jan 1873 in Lonaconing, Allegany Co., MD and died 21 Nov 1945 in Glencoe, Somerset Co., PA. Both are buried in the Mt. Lebanon Reformed Church Cemetery

Children of GEORGE DELOZIER and EMMA PETRY are:

   i. FREDERICK W. DELOZIER (E421)

   ii. ALMA A. DELOZIER (E422)

   iii. MARY M. DELOZIER (E423)

   iv. ALBERT GEORGE DELOZIER (E424) was born in 1906 in Somerset Co., PA.

   v. WALTER GERBER DELOZIER (E425)

   vi. EMMA E. DELOZIER (E426)

   vii. ARTHUR AMERICUS DELOZIER (E427)

   viii. FRANK H. DELOZIER (E428) was born in 1917 in Somerset Co., PA.

Ref: 27-D-GGD-45173, 27-D-EFCP-97224, 9-Larimer Somerset Co PA F49, 10-Northampton Somerset Co PA F50, 11-Northampton Somerset Co PA F70, 44

George G. DeLozier, well known retired hotel keeper, and merchant of Glencoe, died at the home of his daughter, Mrs. J. W. Hartman, in Glencoe, after a lingering illness, on Thursday, May 30th. Funeral services were conducted at the Hartman home at 2:30 p.m., Sunday, by Rev. J. E. Gindlesperger, pastor of the Wills Creek charge of the Reformed Church, followed by interment in the Mt. Lebanon Reformed cemetery, under direction of Johnson & Son, Berlin morticians. The funeral services were largely attended. Floral tributes were many and beautiful. Pallbearers were, W. J. Broadwater, H. C. Cook, H. M. Bittner, M. A. Bittner, H. C. Raupach and C. B. Bittner. Several members of the local church sang an appropriate hymn. Three of his granddaughters from Boswell sang "Sometime We'll Understand" and "Waiting at the Gate". Frank J. Davis, Governor of the Moose Lodge of Cumberland, and Mr. Bowers attended as representatives of that lodge, of which he was a member. Others attending from a distance were Mrs. H. J. Anderson of Glenshaw, Pa.; Mr. and Mrs. F. M. Kunker, Pittsburgh; Mrs. John Dudinack and W. A. DeLozier, Windber; G. W. Petry, Johnstown; Mr. and Mrs. Wm. Petry, Salisbury; G. B. Rhoades and family and A. A. Sharp, Somerset. Mr. DeLozier was aged 69 years and 11 days, having been born in Salisbury, May 19, 1877, a son of Howard and Martha (Bruckman) DeLozier. He grew to manhood in his native town and married Miss Emma Petry of Salisbury, a sister of Frank A. and William R. Petry, prominent building contractors of Salisbury. After his marriage Mr. DeLozier located in Glencoe where he conducted a licensed hotel which did a flourishing business under the Brooks Law until national prohibition made the operation of hotels in small towns unprofitable. After he retired from the hotel business he conducted a general store in Glencoe until his health failed. Mr. and Mrs. DeLozier both were in poor health the last few years, and their children all having grown up and established in homes of their own, the ill and aged parents gave up housekeeping about a year ago and spent their last days in the home of their devoted daughter, Mrs. J. W. Hartman, where Mrs. DeLozier passed away last November 21. Surviving are seven children - Frederick W. and George A. DeLozier, both of Connellsville; Mrs. D. A. Smith, Boswell; Mrs. J. W. Hartman, Glencoe; Walter G., Cumberland, Md.; Mrs. James A. Ludy, Berlin, and Arthur A., Hyndman. He is survived also by two sisters, Mrs. Ada Schrock, Johnstown; Grace DeLozier, Portsmouth, Va., and a brother, W. A. DeLozier, Windber. He left also 21 grandchildren and two great-grandchildren. George DeLozier was a man of affable, kind and generous disposition, devoted to his family and loyal to his friends.   Meyersdale Republican 06 Jun 1946

Emma Petry DeLozier, wife of George G. DeLozier, died at the home of her daughter, Mrs. J. W. Hartman, Glencoe, Pa., Wednesday morning, Nov. 21st, after an illness of almost a year. She was born at Lonaconing, Md., Jan. 21, 1873, and was aged 72 years and 10 months. She was a daughter of Frank and Mary (Walker) Petry. In her infancy her parents moved to Salisbury, Pa., where they lived the remainder of their lives. She grew to womanhood in Salisbury and lived there until her marriage to George G. DeLozier 46 years ago. She is survived by her husband and seven children - Fred W. and G. Albert of Connellsville; Alma, wife of D. A. Smith, Boswell; Mary, wife of J. W. Hartman, Glencoe; W. Gerber, Cumberland; Arthur A., Hyndman, and Emma, wife of James Ludy, Berlin. One son, Frank Howard, preceded her in death by a number of years. Also surviving are two brothers, Frank H. and William A. Petry of Salisbury, 21 grandchildren and two great-grandchildren. Two grandsons, who are serving their country, Chester A. Smith, S 1/c, stationed in the New Hebrides Islands, and 1st Sgt. James E. Hartman, in Atsuga, Japan - could not attend their grandmother's funeral. In her early girlhood she united with the Reformed Church at Salisbury and held her membership there until after taking up her residence in Glencoe in 1910, when she moved her membership to the Glencoe Reformed Church, of which she remained a faithful member always attending Sunday school and church services until her health failed and she was unable to attend. She was also a Charter member of the Ladies Aid Society. Funeral services were conducted Saturday afternoon, Nov. 24th, in the Glencoe Reformed Church at 2 o'clock, by her pastor, Rev. J. E. Gindlesperger. Interment was in the Mt. Lebanon Cemetery, under the direction of Johnson & Son, Berlin morticians.
                     Meyersdale Republican 06 Dec 1945

LUCY MAY DELOZIER was born on 25 Sep 1878 in Somerset Co., PA and died in 07 Apr 1942 in Myersdale, Somerset Co., PA. She married ALLEN ARTHUR SHARP, son of JOSEPH SHARP and ANNA SLOAN. He was born on 19 Oct 1873 in PA and died 30 Nov 1950 in PA. Both are buried in Union Cemetery, Meyersdale, Somerset Co., PA.

Children of LUCY DELOZIER and ALLEN SHARP are:

   i. VESTA F. SHARP (E431)

   ii. ANNIE J. SHARP (E432)

   iii. BLANCHE EVELYN SHARP (E433)

   iv. FAY SHARP (E434) was born in 1920 in Somerset Co., PA.

Ref: 26, 46-D-LMD-40028, 46-D-AAS-96003, 9-Elk Lick Somerset Co PA F150, 10-Laniner Somerset Co PA F15, 44, 54

MRS. LUCY SHARP COMMITS SUICIDE IN ATTIC OF HOME
Meyersdale Woman, 63, Had Been Despondent Due to Ill Health

MEYERSDALE-Mrs. Lucy May (Delozier) Sharp, 63, wife of A. A. Sharp, committed suicide yesterday afternoon by hanging herself in the attic of her home. Discovery of the woman's act was made by her husband after his return home from a nearby garden, where he had been working for more than three hours. Coroner P. S. Dosch said death resulted from strangulation with suicidal intent. The coroner learned that Mrs. Sharp had been in poor health for some time and that she had been very despondent in recent months. The woman used a clothes line in hanging herself. Mrs. Sharp was a daughter of Howard and Martha (Brookman) DeLozier and was born in Somerset County on September 25, 1878. In addition to her husband she is survived by these children; Mrs. J. E. Rhoades, Somerset; Mrs. Charles Henry, Meyersdale, and Mrs. Clyde Housel, Youngstown, O. She also leaves nine grandchildren, an adopted son, Fay Mull, Harrison City, and these brothers and sisters; George G. Delozier, Glencoe; Walter DeLozier, Windber; Mrs. Ada Schrock, Johnstown; and Grace Delozier, residing in the State of Colorado. Funeral services will be conducted at 2:30 o'clock Friday afternoon at the Sharp home. Interment will be in Union Cemetery under the direction of H. R. Konhaus, local mortician.
Johnstown Tribune 08 Apr 1942

Mrs. Lucy May Sharp, aged 64 years, died suddenly at her home on 430 Beachley Street, on Tuesday, April 7, at 3 o'clock p.m. Mrs. Sharp was born in Somerset County on September 25, 1878, a daughter of the late Howard and Martha (Brookman) DeLozier. The deceased, a life-long member of the Lutheran Church, is survived by her husband, A. A. Sharp, and three daughters, Mrs. G. B. Rhodes, of Somerset; Mrs. Charles Henry, of Meyersdale; and Mrs. Claude Housel, of Youngstown, Ohio; one adopted son, Fay Mull, of Harrison City; two brothers, G. G. DeLozier, of Glencoe; and Walter DeLozier, of Windber; two sisters, Mrs. Ada Schrock, of Johnstown, and Grace DeLozier, of Colorado, and nine grandchildren. Services will be conducted at the Sharp home on Beachley Street, on Friday afternoon at 2:30, with Rev. Samuel

Sigler, of Salisbury, in charge. Interment will be made in Union Cemetery under the direction of H. R. Konhaus, local mortician.

Meyersdale Republican 09 Apr 1942

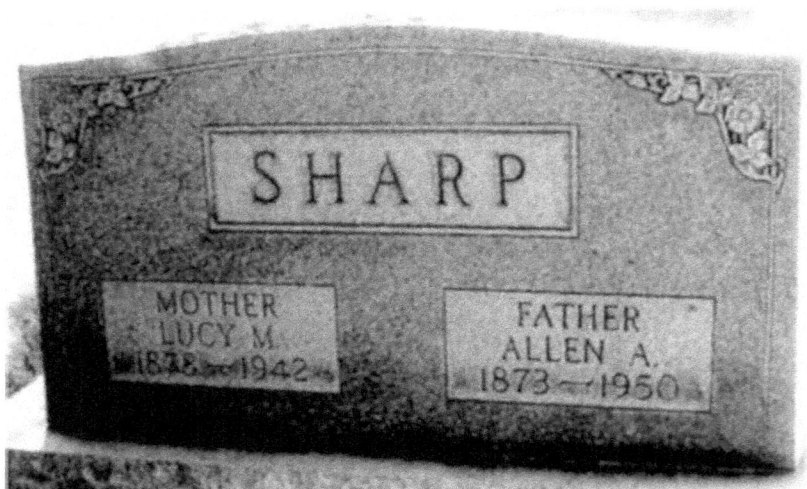

E47 WALTER A. DELOZIER E4

WALTER A. DELOZIER was born in Dec 1884 in Somerset Co., PA and died in 1942 in PA. He married ELIZABETH SMITH, daughter of WHITEMORE SMITH and SUSAN DIEHL. She was born on 23 Jun 1893 in Somerset Co., PA and died 16 Oct 1927 in Johnstown, Cambria Co., PA.

Children of WALTER DELOZIER and ELIZABETH SMITH are:

i. KENNETH MERLE DELOZIER (E471) was born in 17 Sep 1911 in Sand Patch, Somerset Co., PA and died 13 Feb 1973 in Windber, Somerset Co., PA.

Kenneth DeLozier, 61, 1113 Graham Ave., Windber, died Feb. 13, 1973, at home. Born Sept 17, 1911, in Sand Patch, he was a son of the late Walter A. and Elizabeth (Smith) DeLozier. Surviving are these brothers and sisters: Margaret, wife of Theodore Shaw, Uniondale, N.Y.; Mrs. Dorothy Dudinack, Windber; James C., married to the former Norene Moran, Alameda Calif.; and Merle of Buffalo, N.Y. Funeral service was held Friday morning in Marlin G. Meek Funeral Home, Windber, with Rev. Paul Ciampa officiating. Interment in White Oak Cemetery, Meyersdale RD 4.

Meyersdale Republican 22 Feb 1973

ii. MARGARET DELOZIER (E472) was born in 1914 in PA.

iii. DOROTHY MAY DELOZIER (E473) was born on 30 Mar 1916 in Somerset Co., PA and died Jun 1986 in Windber, Somerset Co., PA. She married JOHN DUDINAK on 20 Oct 1934 in Somerset Co., PA, son of JOE DUDINACK and ANNA WOLF. He was born on 19 Aug 1903 in PA and died Jun 1972 in Windber, Somerset Co., PA.

iv. CLAIRE A. DELOZIER (E474) was born in 1919 in PA.

v. JAMES CHARLES DELOZIER (E475)

vi. MERLE DELOZIER (E476)

Ref: 46-D-ES-95894, 10-Ward 1 Scottdale Westmoreland Co PA F91, 12-Ward 4 Windber Somerset Co PA F280, 44, 42, 54, 33

E48 ALICE R. DELOZIER E4

ALICE R. DELOZIER was born on 13 Jan 1887 in Somerset Co., PA and died 09 Apr 1916 in Upper Turkeyfoot Twp., Somerset Co., PA. She married HARVEY LEWIS MULL in Somerset Co., PA. He was born in 1885 in PA and died in 1949 in PA. She is buried in Old Salisbury Cemetery, Salisbury, Somerset Co., PA.

Children of ALICE DELOZIER and HARVEY MULL are:

i. RUTH J. MULL (E481)

ii. PETER HOWARD MULL (E482)

iii. HAZEL ALICE MULL (E483)

iv. SIDNEY FAY MULL (E484)

Ref: 27-D-ARD-3996, 44

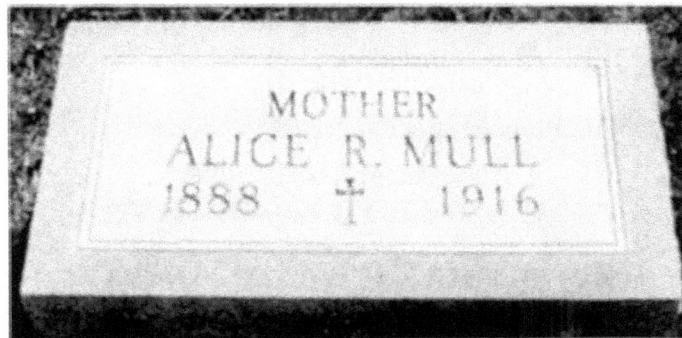

E49 ADA A. DELOZIER E4

ADA A. DELOZIER was born in 13 Jun 1889 in Somerset Co., PA and died in 19 Jul 1972 in PA. She married GEORGE REED SCHROCK. He was born in 1883 in PA and died 1969 in PA. They were divorced 1930-1940. He was married 2nd to EDNA B. DAVIS. Both are buried in Grandview Cemetery, Johnstown, Cambria Co., PA.

Children of ADA DELOZIER and GEORGE SCHROCK are:

i. LEROY P. SCHOCK (E491) was born in 1909 in Bisbee, Cochise Co., AZ and died 1954. He is buried in Grandview Cemetery, Johnstown, Cambria Co., PA.

ii. IDA J. SCHROCK (E492)

iii. THELMA M. SCHROCK (E493) was born on 19 Jan 1915 in Johnstown, Cambria Co., PA and died 23 Jul 1985 in Cambria Co., PA. She married ROBERT THOMAS ELLIS in Johnstown, Cambria Co., PA. He was born on 17 Jun 1914 in PA and died 23 Jul 1985 in Cambria Co., PA. Both are buried in Grandview Cemetery, Johnstown, Cambria Co., PA.

Ref: 26, 9-Ward 3 Bisbee Cochise Co AZ F93, 10-Ward 7 Johnstown Cambria Co PA F86, 11-Johnstown Cambria Co PA F780, 12-Ward 17 Johnstown Cambria Co PA F265, 12-Ward 17 Johnstown Cambria Co PA F266, 44, 42

Mrs. Ada A. Schrock, 83, of 186 Jacob St., Johnstown, died July 19, 1972, at home. Born July 13, 1889, in Salisbury, she was a daughter of Howard and Martha (Brookman) DeLozier, and was the last surviving member of that immediate family. Surviving are two daughters, Mrs. Ida Reese, and Mrs. Thelma Ellis, both of Johnstown, two grandchildren and two great-grandchildren. She was a member of Christ United Methodist Church. Funeral service was held Saturday afternoon in Henderson Funeral Home, Johnstown, with Rev. Howard L. Loveless officiating. Interment in Grandview Cemetery. Attending the funeral were Mr. and Mrs. Arthur DeLozier, Cumberland, Md.; and Mr. and Mrs. John W. Hartman, Glencoe.
Meyersdale Republican 27 July 1972

E211 THOMAS W. ENFIELD E21

Dr. THOMAS W. ENFIELD was born in Jul 1898 in Bedford, Bedford Co., PA. He married CHARLOTTE H. MOORE on 25 Apr 1921 in Philadelphia, Philadelphia Co., PA.

Child of THOMAS ENFIELD and CHARLOTTE is:

i. CHARLOTTE ENFIELD (E2111) was born in Philadelphia, Philidelphia Co., PA.

Ref: 12-Ward 18 Philadelphia Philadelphia Co PA F249

ENFIELD—MOORE

Thomas W. Enfield and Charlotte H. Moore of Llanerch, Pa., were married by Rev. W. C. Kieffer, Monday, April 25, 1921.

The Bedford Gazette 06 May 1921

Announcements were received here this week of the marriage in Philadelphia on Monday of Thomas W. Enfield, eldest son of Dr. and Mrs. Walter F. Enfield of this place, and Miss Charlotte Moore of Llanerch. The young man is a student at the university.

Altoona Tribune 06 May 1921

E212 GEORGE STEWART ENFIELD E21

Dr. GEORGE STEWART ENFIELD was born in 15 May 1900 in Bedford, Bedford Co., PA and died 27 Jan 2000 in Phoenix, Maricopa Co., AZ. He married ROWENA A. ALLMOND, daughter of STELLA E. _____. She was born on 29 Jun 1903 in PA and died Dec 1984 in Scottsdale, Maricopa Co., AZ.

Children of GEORGE ENFIELD and ROWENA ALLMOND are:

  i. STEWART A. ENFIELD (E2121) was born in 1934 in Bedford, Bedford Co., PA.

  ii. GEORGE I. ENFIELD (E2122) was born in 1934 in Bedford, Bedford Co., PA.

Ref: 12-Bedford Bedford Co PA F60, 42

E214 ROBERT FINLEY ENFIELD E21

ROBERT FINLEY ENFIELD was born in 1909 in Bedford, Bedford Co., PA. He married MILDRED H. _____. She was born in 1907 in PA.

Child of ROBERT ENFIELD and MILDRED _____ is:

  i. SAMUEL W. ENFIELD (E2141) was born in 1939 in Bedford, Bedford Co., PA.

Ref: 12-Bedford Bedford Co PA F103

E231 REBECCA ENFIELD E23

REBECCA ENFIELD was born in 1906 in McKeesport, Allegheny Co., PA. She married Dr. CHARLES F. MCDERMOTT, son of C. W. MCDERMOTT.

Child of REBECCA ENFIELD and CHARLES MCDERMOTT is:

  i. CHARLES ENFIELD MCDERMOTT (E2311) was born in 1940 in Pittsburgh, Allegheny Co., PA.

Ref: 12-Ward 28 Pittsburgh Allegheny Co PA F118

Dr. Charles F. McDermott, Pittsburgh dentist, a former resident of Masontown and graduate of German Twp. High School, has been named president-elect of the Pennsylvania Dental Assn.

He is the son of Mr. and Mrs. C. W. McDermott of Masontown and is a 1934 graduate of the University of Pittsburgh's School of Dentistry.

The president-elect is married to the former Rebecca Enfield of Pittsburgh and the couple has one son, Charles F., who will also enter the school of dentistry at Pitt this fall.

Dr. McDermott was elected to the office at the 93rd annual session in Hershey.

He has also served as president of the Odontological Society of Western Pennsylvania and also serves as the society's trustee to the PDA. He is chairman of the PDA Public Information Committee, and is a fellow in the American College of Dentists.

The United States is the largest

The Morning Herald 25 May 1961

E311 PAUL M. STECKMAN E31

PAUL M. STECKMAN was born in 11 Jul 1906 in Altoona, Blair Co., PA and died 21 Sep 1985 in Palm Beach, Palm Beach Co., FL. He married MABEL A. MEARKLE. She was born in 14 Mar 1906 in PA and died 05 Oct 2003 in Palm Beach, Palm Beach Co., FL. Both are buried in Everett Cemetery, Everett, Bedford Co., PA.

Children of PAUL STECKMAN and MABEL MEARKLE are:

i. PATRICIA A. STECKMAN (E3111) was born in 1936 in Butler, Butler Co., PA.

ii. MELBA JEAN STECKMAN (E3112) was born in 1940 in Butler, Butler Co., PA.

Ref: 23-William Richard Griffith, 12-Ward 1 Butler Butler Co PA F350, 42, 26

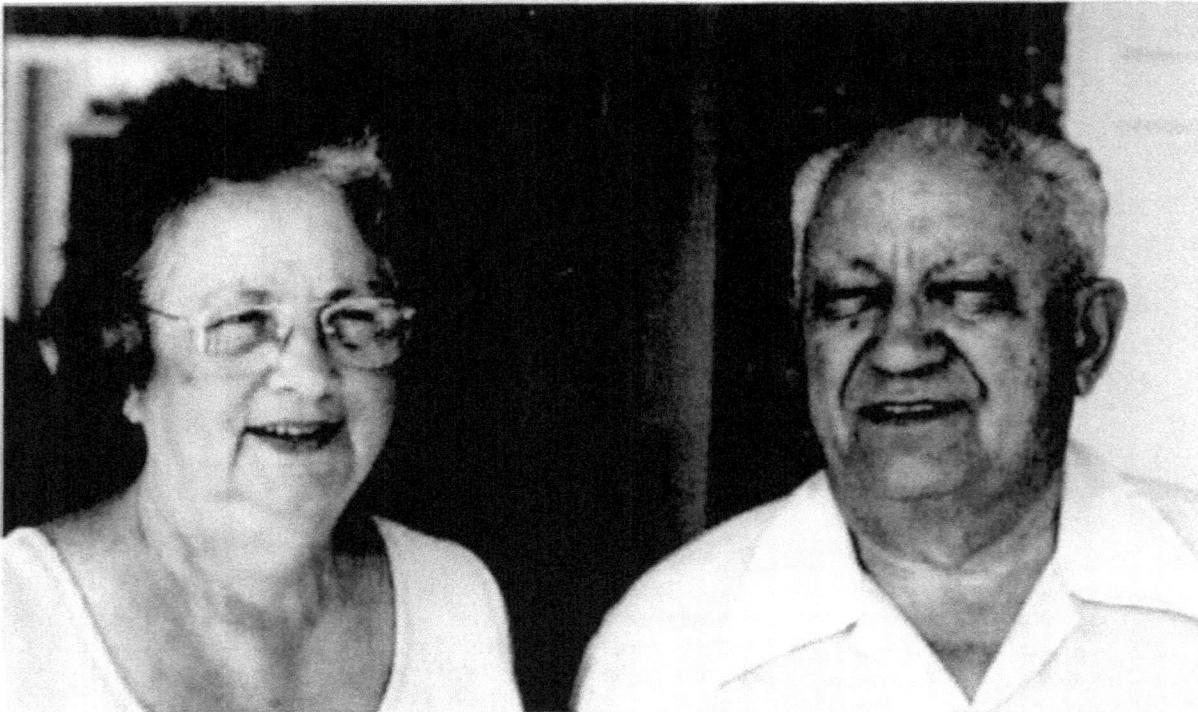

PAUL M. STECKMAN and MABEL A. (MEARKLE) STECKMAN

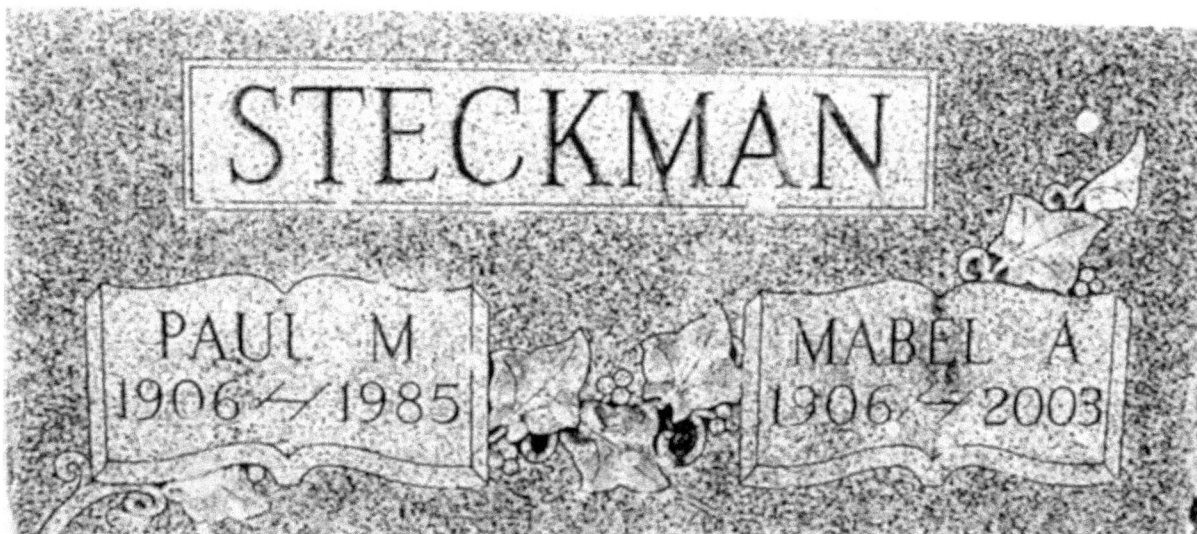

E321 IVAN B. MEANS E32

IVAN B. MEANS was born 1908 in Monroe Twp., Bedford Co., PA. He married VIRGINIA WEIMER. She was born in 1907 in PA.

Children of IVAN MEANS and VIRGINIA WEIMER are:

i. RALPH BRYCE MEANS (E3211)

ii. DORIS MEANS (E3212) was born in 1931 in Bedford Co., PA. She married _____ MUELLER.

iii. LOIS MEANS (E3213) was born in 22 Jul 1931 in Bedford Co., PA. She married _____ HOAGLAND.

iv. RUTH MEANS (E3214) was born in 1936 in Bedford Co., PA. She married _____ BORROR.

v. FLORA GAIL MEANS (E3215)

vi. JOYCE MEANS (E3216) was born on 07 Jul 1945 in Bedford Co., PA. She married JOHN WILLIAM PEPPLE. He was born on 29 Dec 1939.

vii. BLAIR MEANS (E3217) was born and died in infancy in Bedford Co., PA.

Ref: 11-Bedford Bedford Co PA F293, 12-Monroe Twp Bedford Co PA F54, 49

E322 GLADYS R. MEANS E32

GLADYS R. MEANS was born on 24 Oct 1914 in Monroe Twp., Bedford Co., PA and died 14 Feb 2007 in Bedford Co., PA. She married CONDA EARL MILLS. Both are buried in Union Church Cemetery, Clearville, Bedford Co., PA. He was born on 11 Aug 1911 in PA and died 22 Aug 2005 in Bedford Co., PA.

Children of GLADYS MEANS and CONDA MILLS are:

    i. GERALD MILLS (E3221) was born in 1935 in Monroe Twp., Bedford Co., PA

    ii. CLARA E. MILLS (E3222) was born in 1937 in Monroe Twp., Bedford Co., PA

    iii. HELEN A MILLS (E3223) was born in 1939 in Monroe Twp., Bedford Co., PA

Ref: 12-Monroe Twp Bedford Co PA F75, 26

E331 GRANT BRUCKMAN E33

    GRANT BRUCKMAN was born on 17 Feb 1917 in Sproul, Blair Co., PA and died 20 Nov 1984 in Somerset Co., PA. He married MARGARET FRIES.

Children of GRANT BRUCKMAN and MARGARET FRIES are:

    i. BARBARA BRUCKMAN (E3311) married ERIC WILLIAMS.

    ii. ARNOLD BRUCKMAN (E3312)

    iii. ELLEN BRUCKMAN (E3313) married VICTOR SMITH.

    iv. WILLIAM BRUCKMAN (E3314)

Ref: 44

Grant Bruckman, 67, Somerset, died Nov. 20, 1984, at the Masonic Home, Elizabethtown, Pa. Born Feb. 17, 1917, in Sproul, Pa., son of the late Harry and Daisy (Moss) Bruckman. Survived by his wife, the former Margaret Fries; and these children: Mrs. Eric (Barbara) Williams, Arnold, Md.; Mrs. Victor (Ellen) Smith, Fort Lauderdale, Fla.; and William, Somerset; one grandson; and a sister, Mrs. Melvin (Lois) Weyandt, Petersburg, Pa. Arrangements under the direction of the Richard E. Hauger Funeral Home are incomplete. W. Grant Bruckman. Funeral service will be held at 9:30 a.m. Saturday at the Richard E. Hauger Funeral Home, with the Rev. James Vandervort officiating. Interment, Alto Rest Cemetery, Altoona. Friends received 3 to 5 and 7 to 9 p.m. Friday at the funeral Home. Family suggest contributions be made to the Masonic Homes, Elizabethtown, Pa. 17022.
Daily American 23 Nov 1984

E332 LOIS BRUCKMAN E33

    LOIS BRUCKMAN was born on 18 Jun 1920 in Sproul, Blair Co., PA and died 24 Oct 2003 in Huntingdon, Huntingdon Co., PA. She married MELVIN B. WEYANDT on 29 Jun 1940 in Blair Co., PA. He died 13 Mar 2002 in Blair Co., PA.

Children of LOIS BRUCKMAN and MELVIN WEYANDT are:

    i. MIRIAM WEYANDT (E3321) married _____ THOMAS.

ii. PATRICIA WEYANDT (E3322) married _____ ECHARD.

iii. TIMOTHY WEYANDT (E3323) died before 2003.

Ref: 42

E342 KENNETH GIRARD BEASOM E34

KENNETH GIRARD BEASOM was born 08 Jan 1919 in Blair Co., PA and died Apr. 15, 1988 in Altoona, Blair Co., PA. He married JENNIE A. PATTON in Altoona, Blair Co., PA, daughter of J. C. PATTON and ENID G. LEADER. She was born on 01 Jun 1922 in PA. He is buried in Oak Ridge Cemetery, Altoona, Blair Co., PA.

Children of KENNETH BEASOM and JENNIE PATTON are:

i. JEFFREY A. BEASOM (E3421) was born on 16 May 1957.

ii. MICHAEL E. BEASOM (E3422) was born on 01 Sep 1962.

iii. GARRETT A. BEASOM (E3423) was born on 01 Sep 1962.

iv. SAMANTHA G. BEASOM (E3424) was born on 10 Oct 1973.

Ref: 42, 49

Local Officer Returns to Army Post

1st Lt. Kenneth G. Beasom, 26, son of Mrs. B. E. Coltobaugh, 1509 Crawford avenue, arrived in Miami Beach, Fla., this week after spending a 21-day furlough in Altoona. He was accompanied to Florida by his wife, the former Jennie Patton, 1500 Crawford avenue.

Lt. Beasom completed 35 missions over enemy-held territory, as the pilot of a B-17 Flying Fortress of the 8th AAF based in England. He is authorized to wear the Air medal, to which has been added five Oak Leaf clusters. Going overseas as a second lieutenant, he was promoted to his present rank at the air base. Although uninjured by the heavy enemy fire encountered on many missions, he reports that sixty-four flak holes were coounted on his plane after one trip.

The lieutenant has been assigned to the air transport command with headquarters in New York city.

A graduate of the Altoona High school, he was formerly employed by the Wm. F. Gable Co., and the Juniata shops of the Pennsylvania railroad.

Altoona Tribune 16 Apr 1945

U.S. World War II Army Enlistment Records, 1938-1946

Name: Kenneth G Beasom
Birth Year: 1919
Race: White, citizen (White)
Nativity State or Country: Pennsylvania
State of Residence: Pennsylvania
County or City: Blair
Enlistment Date: 10 Dec 1941
Enlistment State: Pennsylvania
Enlistment City: New Cumberland
Branch: Branch Immaterial - Warrant Officers, USA
Branch Code: Branch Immaterial - Warrant Officers, USA
Grade: Private
Grade Code: Private
Term of Enlistment: Enlistment for the duration of the War or other emergency, plus six months, subject to the discretion of the President or otherwise according to law
Component: Selectees (Enlisted Men)
Source: Civil Life
Education: 4 years of high school
Civil Occupation: Electricians
Marital Status: Married
Height: 70
Weight: 128

COMMONWEALTH OF PENNSYLVANIA
WORLD WAR II VETERANS' COMPENSATION BUREAU

APPLICATION FOR WORLD WAR II COMPENSATION—TO BE USED BY HONORABLY DISCHARGED VETERAN OR PERSON STILL IN SERVICE

MAR 22 1950

IMPORTANT—Before Filling Out This Form Study it Carefully.
Read and Follow Instructions—Print Plainly in Ink or Use Typewriter. DO NOT Use Pencil—All Signatures Must Be in Ink.

Applicant Must Not Write In Space Below

MAR 11 1950
Date Application Was Received

1—Name of Applicant.
Beasom   Kenneth   G.
Last   First   Middle or Initial

Batch Control Number
7248

2—Address to Which CHECK and MAIL is to be Sent.
1500 Crawford Ave. Ahtoona Blair Pa.
House No. St. R. D. P. O. Box   City or Town   County   State

Active Domestic Service
Months 34 $ 340
Days $
Amount Due $ 340

3—Date and Place of Birth.
Jan. 8 1919 Ahtoona Blair Pa.
Month Day Year City or Town County State

Active Foreign Service
Months 8 $ 120
Days $
Amount Due $ 120

4—Name Under Which Applicant Served In World War II.
Same Name
Last   First   Middle or Initial

Total Amt. Due $ 460

5—Date of Beginning and Date of Ending of Each Period of Service Between December 7, 1941 and March 2, 1946 (Both Dates Inclusive) During Which Applicant Was In DOMESTIC SERVICE.
Dec. 10, 1941   30 - 43   July 21, 1944
March 16, 1945   2 - 23   June 7, 1945
Date of Beginning   Date of Ending

Audited By
Service Computed By
Amounts Extended By

6—Date of Beginning and Date of Ending of Each Period of Service Between December 7, 1941 and March 2, 1946 (Both Dates Inclusive) During Which Applicant Was In FOREIGN SERVICE.
July 22, 1944   7 - 25   March 15, 1945
Date of Beginning   Date of Ending

MAR 20 1950
Date
For A. G.
For Aud. G.
For S. T.
Application Disapproved
By

7—Date and Place Applicant Entered Active Service.
Dec. 10 1941 New Cumberland, Pa.
Month Day Year Place

8—Service or Serial Numbers Assigned To Applicant.
Service No's.
Serial No's. 33177743 / 0-821144

9—Date and Place Where Applicant Was Separated From Active Service.
June 7 1945 Fort Dix, New Jersey
Month Day Year Place

10—Is Applicant Now Serving In Armed Forces On Active Duty? Yes _____ No No
If Answer is YES—Be Sure To Have Certificate Executed And Filed With Application—See Instruction Sheet.

11—Mark "X" Above Name To Indicate Sex And Branch of Service.
X   X
Male Female Army Navy Marine Corps Coast Guard Other—Describe

12—Applicant's Residence At Time of Entry Into Active Service.
1500 Crawford Ave.   Ahtoona Blair Pa.
House No. Street R. D. P. O. Box City or Town County State

13—Applicant Was Registered Under Selective Service As Follows.
3   Ahtoona Blair Pa.
Draft Board No. City or Town County State

E351 DANIEL ALBERT BRUCKMAN E35

DANIEL ALBERT BRUCKMAN was born on 12 Mar 1917 in Altoona, Blair Co., PA and died 08 Jan 1996 in Altoona, Blair Co., PA He married JOSEPHINE LOUISE BROWN on 01 Jan 1951 in Corsica, Jefferson Co., PA, daughter of CHARLES WILLIAM BROWN and ESTHER LOLA SMALL. She was born on 04 Jul 1921 in Corsica, Jefferson Co., PA and died 13 Dec 2013 in Altoona, Blair Co., PA. Both are buried at the Alto-Reste Park Cemetery,

Altoona, Blair Co., PA. On 10 Dec 1941, he enlisted at New Cumberland, PA as a Private US Army to serve in WW II. He served as a rank of T-3 in the Army Medic 834 Engineer Aviation Battalion and on 07 Jun 1944, Landed in France D-Day +1.

Child of DANIEL BRUCKMAN and JOSEPHINE BROWN is:

   i. ESTHER MAY BRUCKMAN (E3511)

Ref: 47, 48

Josephine L. Bruckman July 4, 1921 – Dec. 13, 2013

Josephine L. Bruckman, 92, Altoona, went home to be with the Lord late Friday morning at Valley View Health and Rehabilitation Center. She was born in Corsica, Pa., daughter of the late Charles and Esther (Small) Brown. She married Daniel A. Bruckman on Jan. 1, 1951, in Corsica. He preceded her in death on Jan. 8, 1996.Surviving are a daughter, Esther M. Brooks and her husband, Duane, of Altoona; three granddaughters: Rebecca Brooks in North Carolina, Rachel Brooks in Kansas and Ruth Brooks in Georgia; a brother, Charles Brown in North Carolina; and a sister, Emma Jean Howell in New York. Josephine was preceded in death by a brother, John Brown; and two sisters: Betty Brown and Winifred Haugh. Josephine was a graduate of Corsica Union High School and Philadelphia School of the Bible. She was a homemaker and a member of Calvary Baptist Church, Altoona, where she enjoyed working with children. Friends will be received from 6 to 8 p.m. Tuesday, Dec. 17, 2013, and 10 to 11 a.m. Thursday, Dec. 19, 2013, at Myers-Somers Funeral Home Inc., 501 Sixth Ave., Altoona, where a funeral service will be held at 11 a.m. Thursday Dec. 19, 2013, with Pastor Larry Weaver officiating. Interment will be made at Alto-Reste Park Cemetery. In remembrance of Josephine, memorial contributions may be made to Calvary Baptist Church, Missions Fund, 810 Ruskin Drive, Altoona, PA 16602.

The Altoona Mirror 15 Dec 2013

U.S. World War II Army Enlistment Records, 1938-1946

Name: Daniel A Bruckman
Birth Year: 1917
Race: White, citizen (White)
Nativity State or Country: Pennsylvania
State of Residence: Pennsylvania
County or City: Blair
Enlistment Date: 10 Dec 1941
Enlistment State: Pennsylvania
Enlistment City: New Cumberland
Branch Code: Branch Immaterial - Warrant Officers, USA
Grade: Private
Grade Code: Private
Term of Enlistment: Enlistment for the duration of the War or other emergency, plus six months, subject to the discretion of the President or otherwise according to law
Component: Selectees (Enlisted Men)
Source: Civil Life
Education: 4 years of high school
Civil Occupation: Salespersons
Marital Status: Single, without dependents
Height:68
Weight: 126

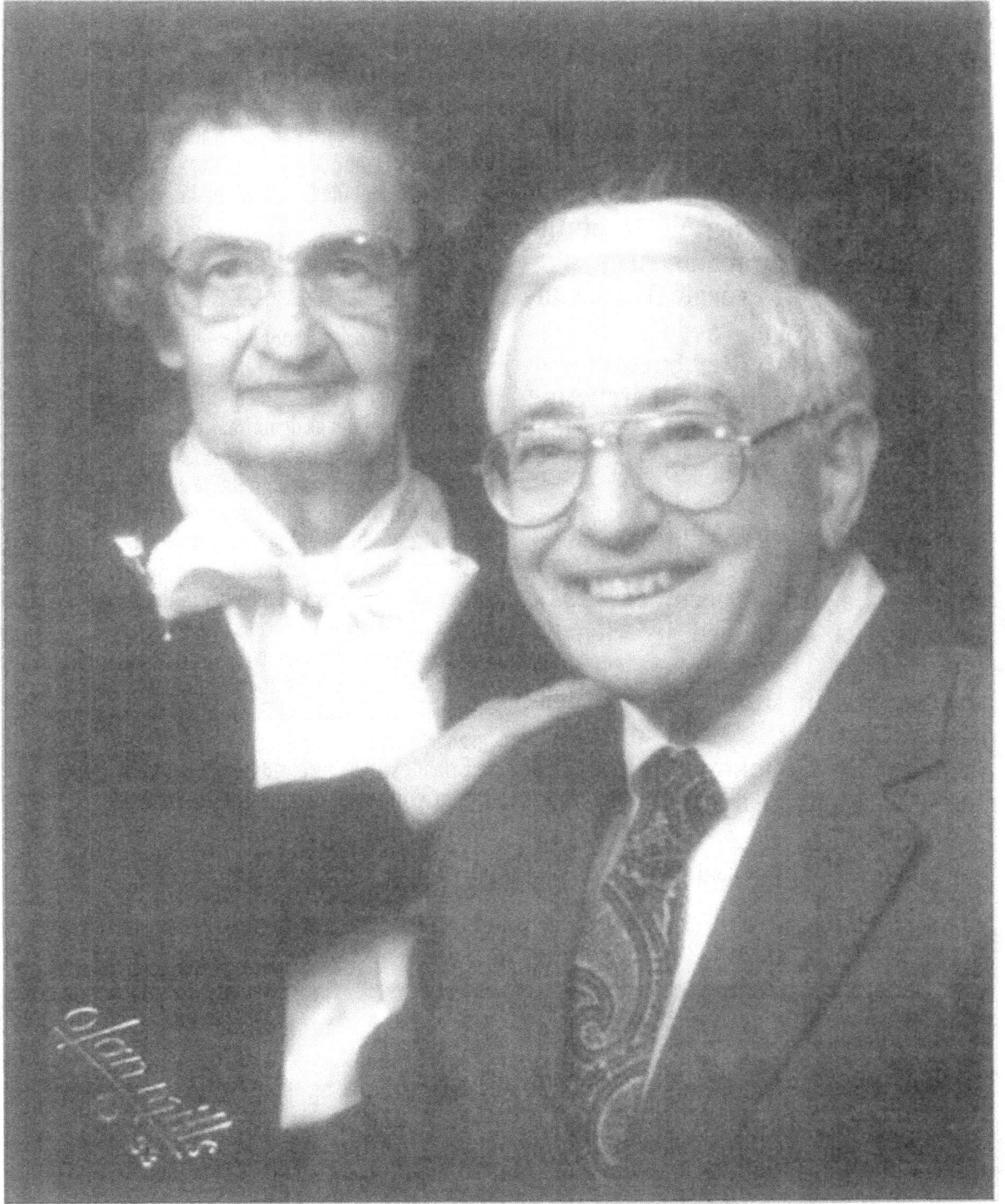

DANIEL ALBERT and JOSEPHINE LOUISE (BROWN) BRUCKMAN

Technician Fifth Grade Daniel A. Bruckman of Altoona and Private First Class Leo A. Brown of Greenwood, have completed 32 months of overseas service with the 834th Engineer Aviation battalion which has just been released from the censor's secret list along with other units of the IX Engineer Command.

Bruckman, a surgical technician,, and Brown, a duty soldier, are serving with the battalion in Germany where it is constructing front-line airfields for tactical air-ground operations of the U. S. Ninth Air force.

A graduate of Altoona Senior High school, Bruckman entered the service in December 1941. Brown was employed by Schaeffers bakery before he entered the service in June 1942. Bruckman's parents, Mr. and Mrs. Charles H. Bruckman, live at 1423 Washington avenue.

Rev. Daniel A. Bruckman

The Rev. Daniel A. Bruckman, 78, Logan Hills Apartments, died Monday afternoon, Jan. 8, 1996, at Van Zandt VA Medical Center, following an extended illness.

He was born March 12, 1917, in Altoona, the son of Charles H. and Mary (Detwiler) Bruckman. He married Josephine L. Brown on Jan. 1, 1951, in Corsica.

Rev. Bruckman was a member of Calvary Baptist Church.

He pastored at Mountaindale Baptist Church, Fairview Chapel, Altoona, Berean Bible Fellowship, Clymer, and South Altoona Baptist Church. He also taught at the Altoona Bible Institute for 29 years, and served as dean from 1977 to 1982. He also worked as a painter.

Rev. Bruckman was a graduate of Altoona High School and Altoona Bible Institute and a 1949 graduate of Philadelphia School of Bible.

He was an Army veteran of World War II.

Rev. Bruckman was a member of the Independent Fundamental Churches of America.

Surviving are his wife, a daughter, Esther M. Brooks of Altoona; a brother, Philip E. of Coplay; a sister, Doris F. Lantz of Pensacola, Fla.; and three grandchildren.

Friends will be received from 1 to 4 p.m. Thursday at William G. Bigelow II Funeral Home.

Altoona Tribune 02 May 1945   Altoona Mirror 10 Jan 1996

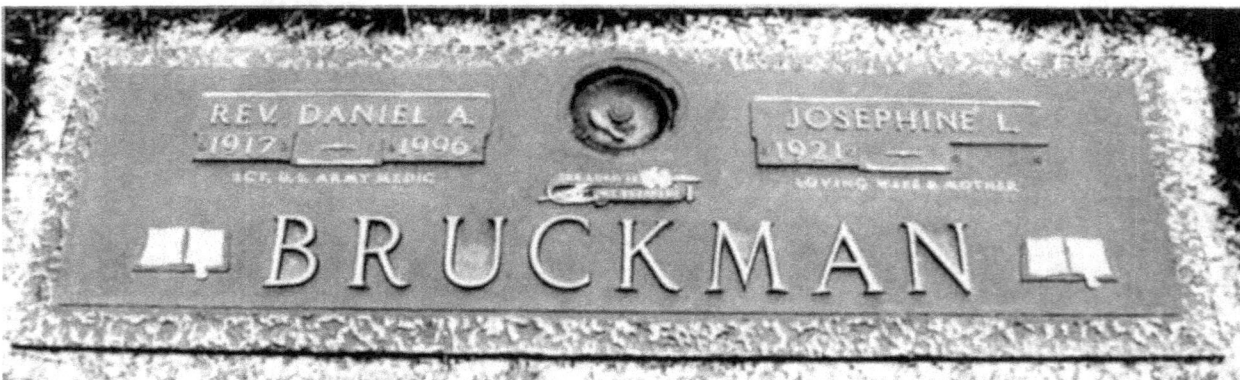

REV DANIEL A. 1917 - 1996   SGT. U.S. ARMY MEDIC   JOSEPHINE L. 1921 -   LOVING WIFE & MOTHER   BRUCKMAN

Form No. 1 ⟨⟩—10

COMMONWEALTH OF PENNSYLVANIA
WORLD WAR II VETERANS' COMPENSATION BUREAU

APPLICATION FOR WORLD WAR II COMPENSATION—TO BE USED BY HONORABLY DISCHARGED VETERAN OR PERSON STILL IN SERVICE

IMPORTANT—Before Filling Out This Form Study it Carefully.

Read and Follow Instructions—Print Plainly in Ink or Use Typewriter. DO NOT Use Pencil—All Signatures Must Be in Ink.

		Applicant Must Not Write In Space Below
		FEB 10 1950
		Date Application Was Received
		Batch Control Number
		2689

1—Name of Applicant.

BRUCHMAN   DANIEL   ALBERT

Last   First   Middle or Initial

Active Domestic Service	
Months 8	$ 80
Days	$
Amount Due $	80

2—Address to Which CHECK and MAIL is to be Sent.

1423 Washington Avenue   Altoona,   Blair   Pa.

House No. St. R. D. P. O. Box   City or Town   County   State

Active Foreign Service	
Months 38	$
Days	$ 420.
Amount Due $	

3—Date and Place of Birth.

March 12, 1917   Altoona   Blair   Pa.

Month   Day   Year   City or Town   County   State

Total Amt. Due $ 500.00

4—Name Under Which Applicant Served In World War II.

Same Name

Last   First   Middle or Initial

Audited By _____

Service Computed By _____

5—Date of Beginning and Date of Ending of Each Period of Service Between December 7, 1941 and March 2, 1946 (Both Dates Inclusive) During Which Applicant Was In DOMESTIC SERVICE.

10 December 1941   to   5 Aug. 1942

Oct. 3, 1945   6-5   Oct. 7, 1945

Date of Beginning   Date of Ending

Amounts Extended By _____

Date FEB 22 1950

For A. G. _____

6—Date of Beginning and Date of Ending of Each Period of Service Between December 7, 1941 and March 2, 1946 (Both Dates Inclusive) During Which Applicant Was In FOREIGN SERVICE.

5 August 1942   to   2 October 1945

37-29

Date of Beginning   Date of Ending

For Aud. G. _____

7—Date and Place Applicant Entered Active Service.

Dec. 10, 1941   New Cumberland, Pa.

Month   Day   Year   Place

For S. T. _____

Application Disapproved

By _____

8—Service or Serial Numbers Assigned To Applicant.

Service No's. _____

Serial No's. 33117784

9—Date and Place Where Applicant Was Separated From Active Service.   Indiantown Gap, Pa.

October 7, 1945   Unit B Sep. Center 45 IGMR Pa.

Month   Day   Year   Place

10—Is Applicant Now Serving In Armed Forces On Active Duty?   Yes _____   No   No

If Answer Is YES—Be Sure To Have Certificate Executed And Filed With Application—See Instruction Sheet.

11—Mark "X" Above Name To Indicate Sex And Branch of Service.

X   X

Male   Female   Army   Navy   Marine Corps   Coast Guard   Other—Describe

12—Applicant's Residence At Time of Entry Into Active Service.

1423 Washington Ave.   Altoona,   Blair   Pa.

House No.   Street   R. D.   P. O. Box   City or Town   County   State

13—Applicant Was Registered Under Selective Service As Follows.

LOCAL BOARD #2   ALTOONA   BLAIR   PA.

Draft Board No.   City or Town   County   State

PAUL RAYMOND BRUCKMAN was born on 10 Aug 1922 in Altoona, Blair Co., PA and died 24 Feb 1992 in Eldorado, Blair Co., PA. He married (1) MARY AUTHALIA AVERY on 26 Aug 1944 in Corinth, Alcorn Co., MS, daughter of MARVIN E. AVERY and ANNIE A. MORRIS. She was born 10 Sep 1927 in Crockett Co., TN and died 20 Oct 2010 in Jackson, Madison Co., TN. They were divorced in 1965. He married (2) ARTIMESIA M. BUTTERBAUGH on 14 Jun 1971 in Altoona, Blair Co., PA. She was born on 19 Aug 1923 in Altoona, Blair Co., PA and died 24 Aug 1984 in Lancaster, Lancaster Co., PA. He is buried in Alto-Reste Park Cemetery. He served in the US Army in WW II as Tech 4. His 2nd wife buried in Rose Hill Cemetery, Altoona, Blair Co., PA.

Children of PAUL BRUCKMAN and MARY AVERY are:

  i. GERALD THOMAS BRUCKMAN (E3531)

  ii. RANDALL EUGENE BRUCKMAN (E3532)

Ref: 49, 42, 23-Raymond Clyde Lantz, 12-Civil District 8 Crockett Co TN H4, 74, 23-Randall Eugene Bruckman

BRUCKMAN—AVERY

Mr. and Mrs. C. H. Bruckman of 1423 Washington avenue announce the marriage of their son, Pfc. Paul Raymond Bruckman of Camp Crowder, Mo., to Miss Mary Authalia Avery, daughter of Mr. and Mrs. Marvin E. Avery of Alamo, Tenn. The ceremony was performed on Saturday, Aug. 26, in Corinth, Miss. The couple is residing at 605 North High street, Neosho, Mo.

Altoona Mirror 25 Sep 1944

Paul R. Bruckman, member of a signal training regiment at Camp Crowder, Mo., has been promoted to private first class and is now taking a radio operator high speed course at the signal corps school. He is a son of Mr. and Mrs. Charles H. Bruckman, 1423 Washington avenue. He was inducted in December, 1942.

Altoona Tribune 21 Oct 1943

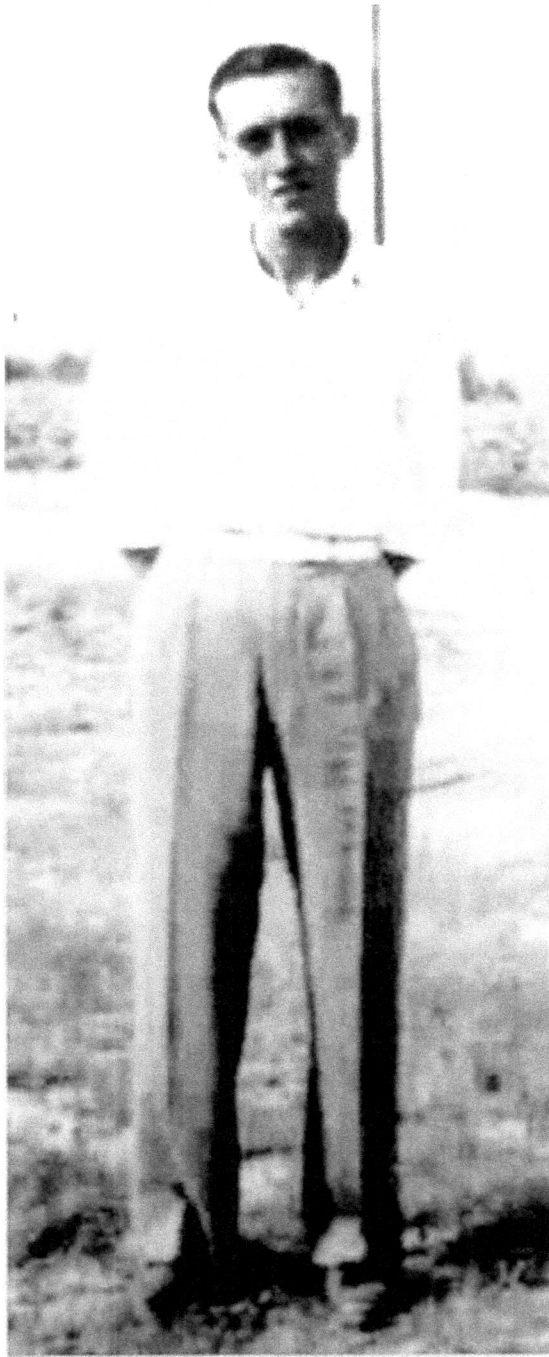

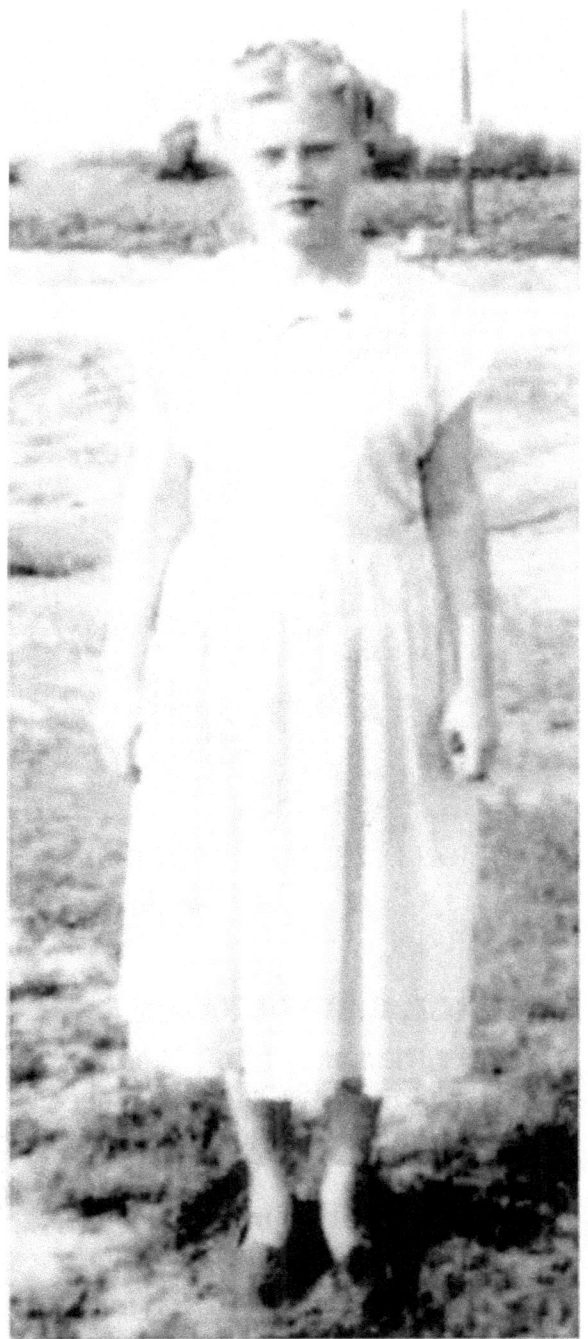

PAUL RAYMOND and MARY AUTHALIA (AVERY) BRUCKMAN

MARY A. McARTHUR, 83, died October 20, 2010. Visitation for Mrs. McArthur will be 12-2 p.m. Friday, October 22, at Ronk Funeral Home. Funeral services to follow at 2 p.m. in the chapel of the funeral home. Interment will follow in Cairo Cemetery. Mrs. McArthur was preceded in death by her daughter, Lisa Kinsey; grandson, Cameron Kinsey. Surviving relatives include her sons, Jerry Bruckman and wife Sandy, Randy Bruckman and wife Pam; daughter, Donna Richardson and friend Tim; 11 grandchildren; 10 great-grandchildren. Ronk Funeral Home Alamo, TN 731-696-5555

The Commercial Appeal 21 Oct 2010

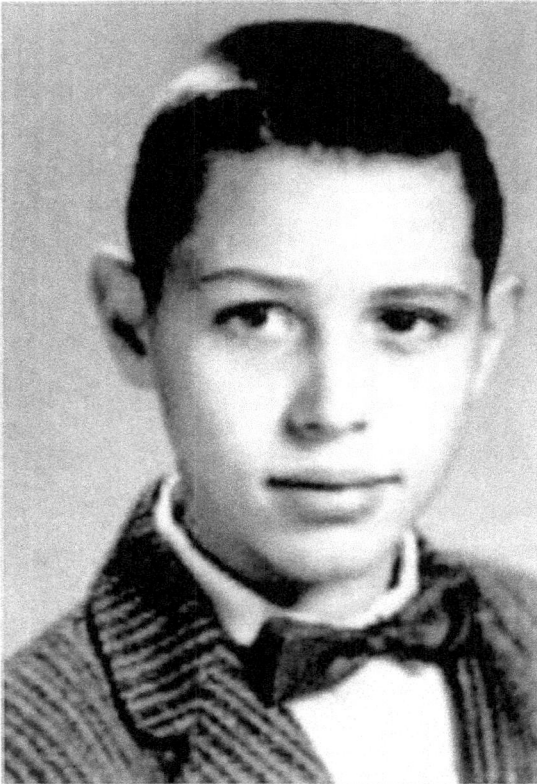
GERALD THOMAS BRUCKMAN

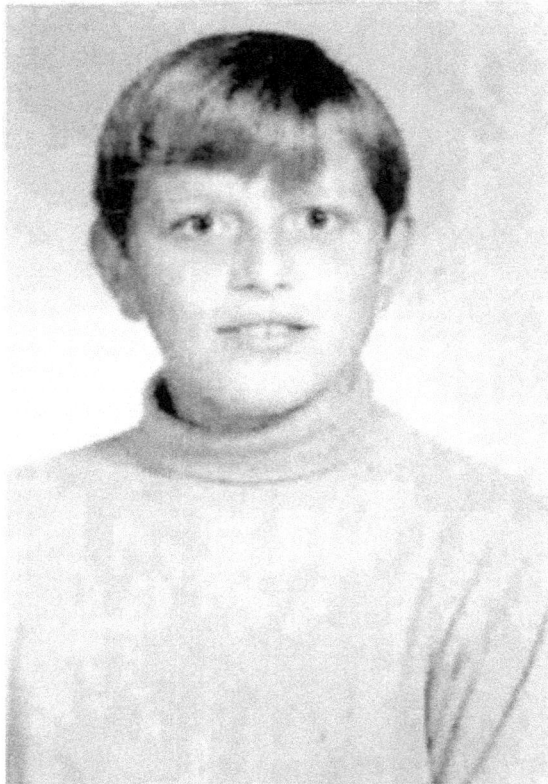
RANDALL EUGENE BRUCKMAN

PAUL R. BRUCKMAN

Mr. Bruckman, 69, of Eldorado Mobile Home Court died unexpectedly at 10 p.m. Monday, Feb. 24, 1992, at home.

Mr. Bruckman retired as a civil service computer technician.

He was born Aug. 10, 1922, in Altoona, the son of Charles H. and Mary I. (Detwiler) Bruckman. He married Artimesia Butterbaugh on June 14, 1971, in Altoona. She preceded him in death.

Surviving are two sons: Gerald T. of Southaven, Miss., and Randall E. of Bartlett, Tenn.; and seven grandchildren.

Also surviving are three brothers and a sister: the Rev. Daniel A. and Doris Lantz of Altoona, Philip E. of Coplay and Harold H.

Mr. Bruckman attended Calvary Baptist Church.

He was an Army veteran of World War II.

Mr. Bruckman was a 1941 graduate of Altoona High School.

Friends will be received from 7 to 9 p.m. Thursday at William G. Bigelow Funeral Home.

Altoona Mirror 26 Feb 1992

90

PAUL R BRUCKMAN
TEC 4   US ARMY
WORLD WAR II
AUG 10 1922   FEB 24 1992

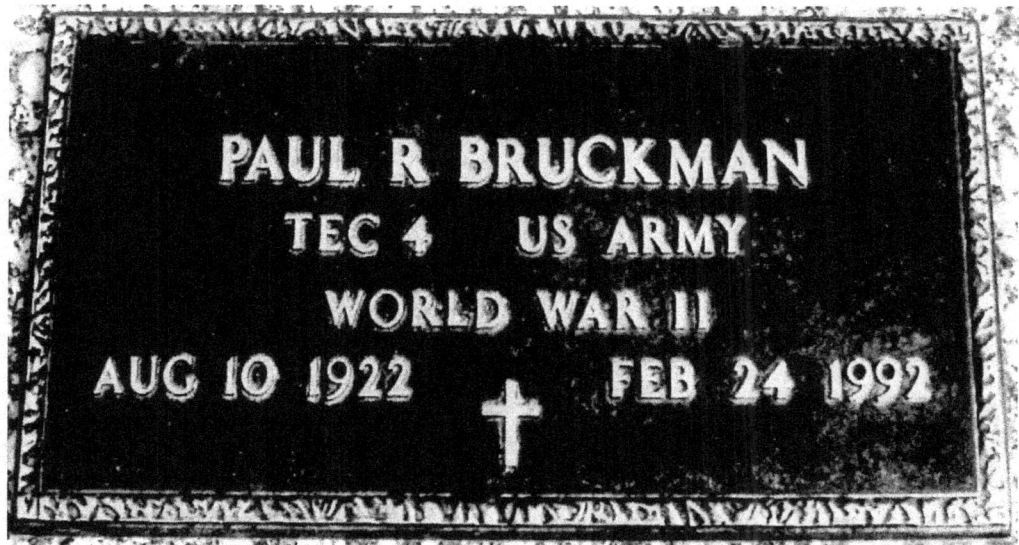

E355 DORIS FAYE BRUCKMAN E35

DORIS FAYE BRUCKMAN was born 02 Oct 1930 in Altoona, Blair Co., PA, and died 11 Feb 2004 in Pensacola, Escambia Co., FL. She married RAYMOND GARFIELD LANTZ on 12 Jan 1951 in Winchester, Frederick Co., VA, son of CLYDE RAYMOND LANTZ and CATHERINE WILNORA GOOD. He was born on 29 Jul 1929 in Altoona, Blair Co., PA, and died 11 Mar 2006 in Altoona, Blair Co., PA. He served in the U.S. Navy 12 Sep 1946-21 Feb 1950, on 13 Aug 1946, enlisted at Pittsburgh, PA, on 15 May 1949, advanced to rank of AM3 and on 21 Feb 1950, was honorably discharged at NAS Key West, FL. He was a bartender most of 1955-1979 at various establishments in Altoona, Blair Co., PA, an electronic repair technician for a short time during that period and finally in 1980 was from 1980, Owner & Operator of Ray's Handy Store till he retired. She was a nurse's aide 1961-1968 Altoona Hospital, Altoona, Blair Co., PA and in 1970 Laundry Worker, Penn Alto Hotel, Altoona, Blair Co., PA for a number of years until retired.

Child of DORIS BRUCKMAN and RAYMOND LANTZ is:

   i. RAYMOND CLYDE LANTZ (E3551)

Ref: 24, 25, 27-B/DFB/154546/DOC PA, 27-D/DFL/14946309/Escambia Co FL, 27-B/RGL/1041310-1929/DOH PA, 27-D/RGL/P12307661/DOH PA, 27-M/RGL&DFB/1819310/DOH VA

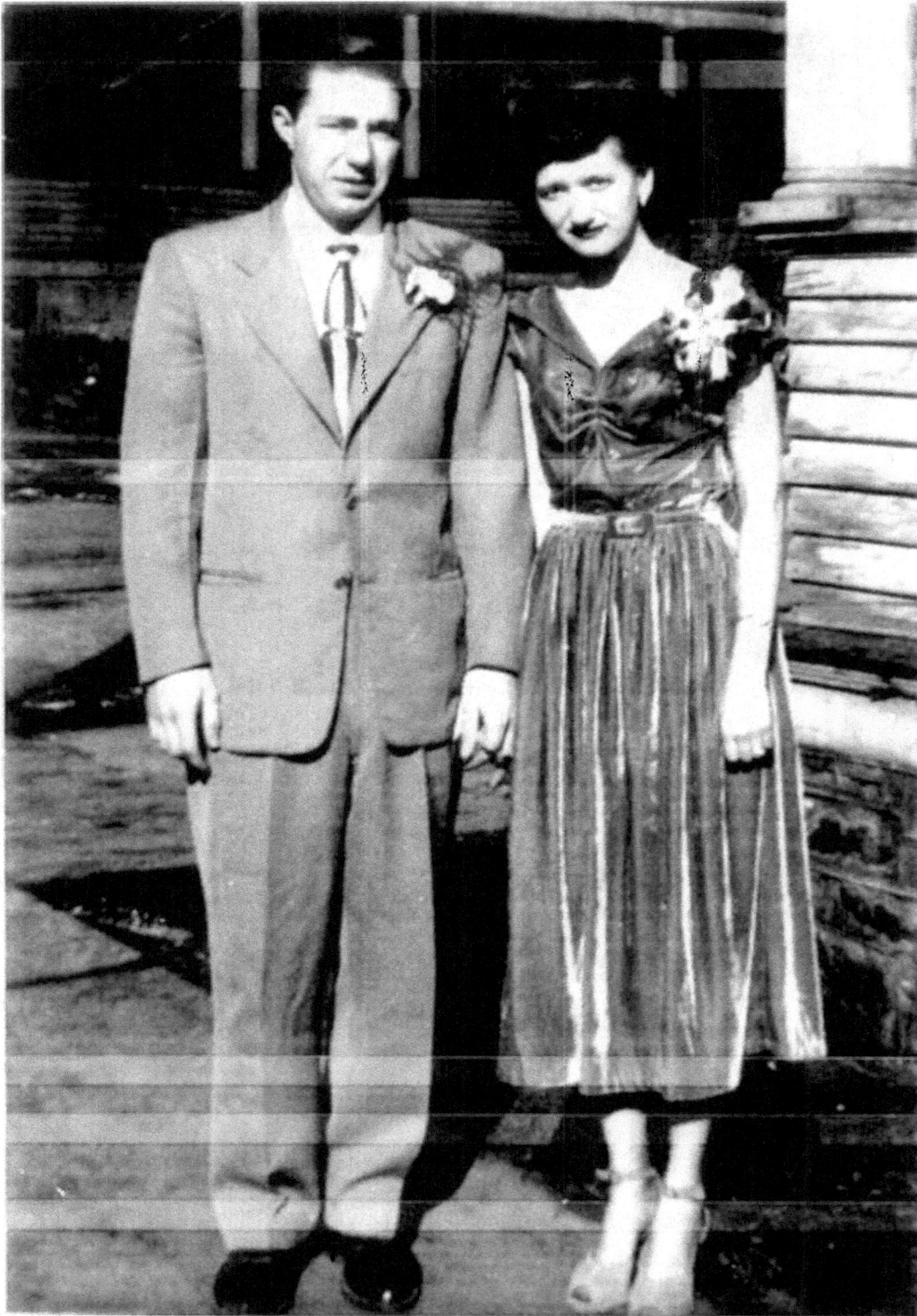

RAYMOND GARFIELD and DORIS FAYE (BRUCKMAN) LANTZ

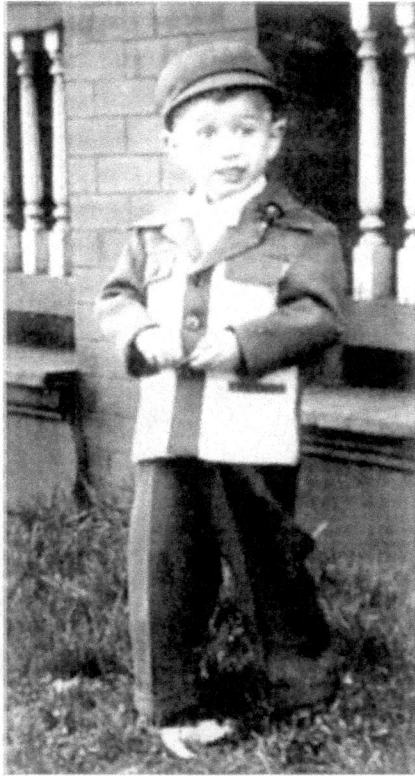
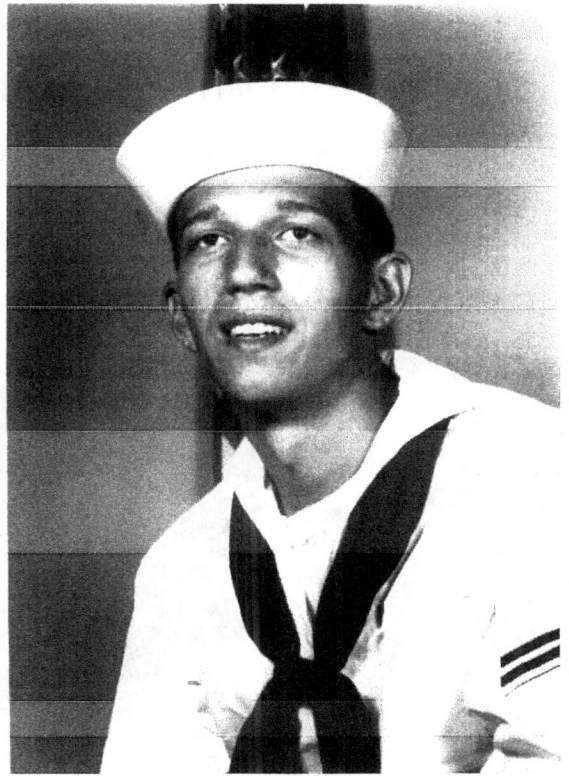

RAYMOND CLYDE LANTZ

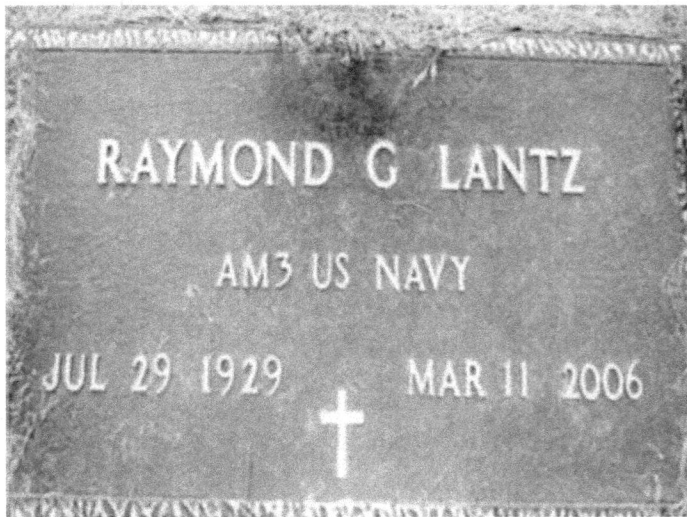

RAYMOND G LANTZ

AM3 US NAVY

JUL 29 1929   MAR 11 2006

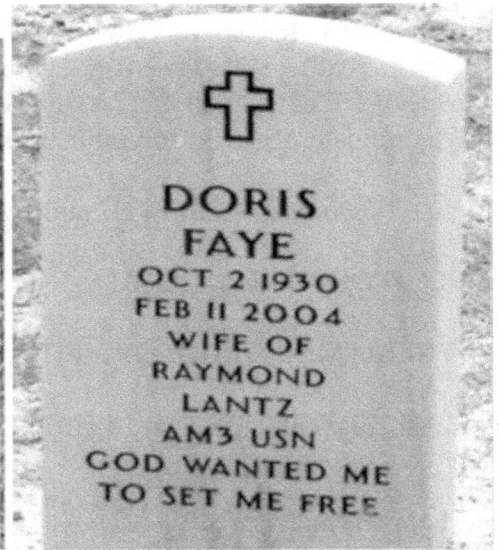

DORIS
FAYE
OCT 2 1930
FEB 11 2004
WIFE OF
RAYMOND
LANTZ
AM3 USN
GOD WANTED ME
TO SET ME FREE

E361 ROBERT RALPH GRIFFITH E36

ROBERT RALPH GRIFFITH was born on 20 Apr 1916 in Altoona, Blair Co., PA and died 12 Mar 2004 in Seattle, King Co., WA. He married JEAN LUEKE. She was born on 27 Nov 1924 He is buried in Sunset Hills Memorial Park, Bellevue, King Co., WA.

Children of ROBERT GRIFFITH and JEAN LUEKE are:

   i. GREG GRIFFITH (E3611) married ANITA _____.

   ii. GARY GRIFFITH (E3612) married DONNA _____.

   iii. LORI GRIFFITH (E3613) married STEVE BARNARD.

Ref: 52, 23-William Richard Griffith

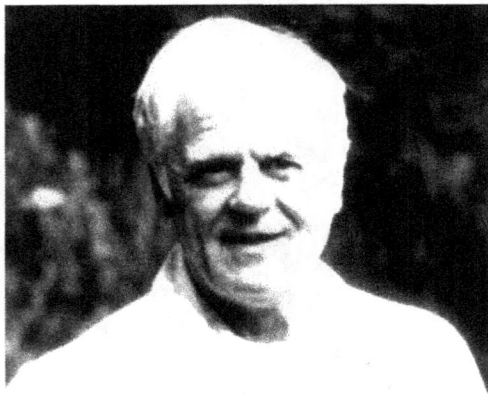

ROBERT R. GRIFFITH

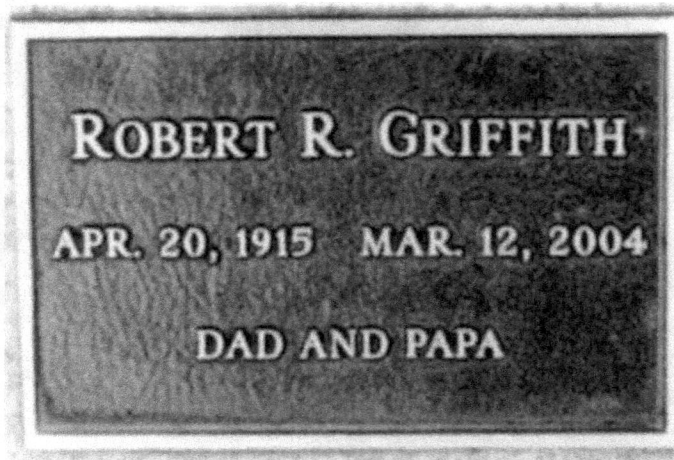

E362 DONALD RICHARD GRIFFITH E36

    DONALD RICHARD GRIFFITH was born on 30 Jan 1917 in Blair Co., PA and died 22 Dec 2006 in Seattle, King Co., WA. He married JEAN MARIAN ROBERTSON, daughter of JAMES ROBERTSON and ELIZABETH MACHIE GORDON. She was born in 13 Dec 1918 in New Westminister, British Columbia, Canada and died 02 Feb 1996 in Seattle, King Co., WA.

Children of DONALD GRIFFITH and JEAN ROBERTSON are:

   i. PEGGY GRIFFITH (E3621)

   ii. WILLIAM RICHARD GRIFFITH (E3622)

Ref: 53, 42, 23-William Richard Griffith

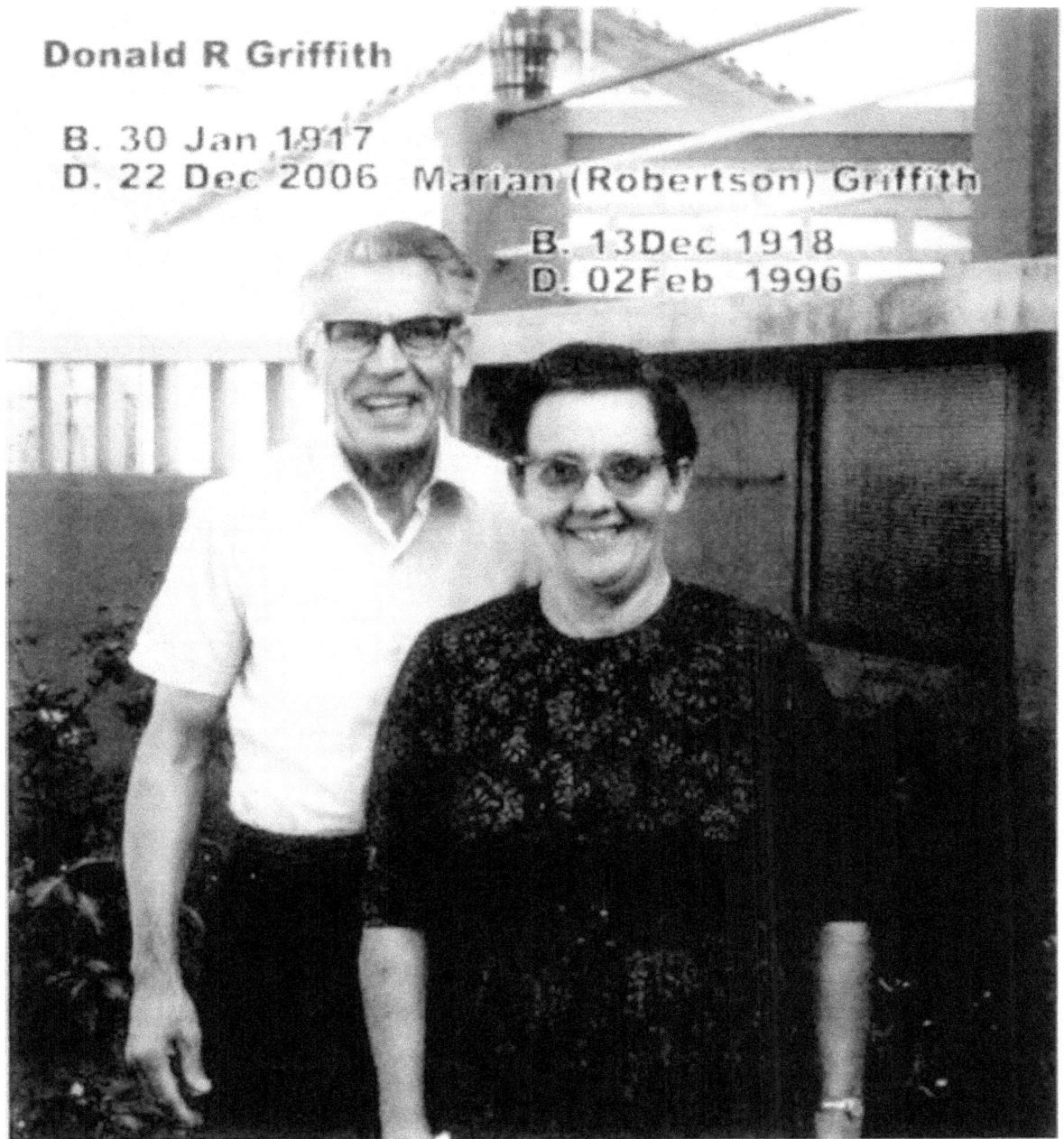

Donald R Griffith

B. 30 Jan 1917
D. 22 Dec 2006   Marian (Robertson) Griffith

B. 13 Dec 1918
D. 02 Feb 1996

E363 ARTHUR RAYMOND GRIFFITH E36

ARTHUR RAYMOND GRIFFITH was born on 18 Sep 1921 in Blair Co., PA and died 13 Sep 2006 in Edinburg, Hidalgo Co., TX. He married SHIRLEY MAE AFRICA. She was born on 15 Mar 1926 and died 11 Apr 2008. Both are buried in Fort Sam Houston National Cemetery, San Antonio, Bexar Co., TX.

Children of ARTHUR GRIFFITH and SHIRLEY AFRICA are:

i. SUSAN GRIFFITH (E3631)

ii. CHRISTINE GRIFFITH (E3632) married _____ RITCHEY.

Form No. 1 ~~~~10

COMMONWEALTH OF PENNSYLVANIA
WORLD WAR II VETERANS' COMPENSATION BUREAU

APPLICATION FOR WORLD WAR II COMPENSATION—TO BE USED BY HONORABLY DISCHARGED VETERAN OR PERSON STILL IN SERVICE

IMPORTANT—Before Filling Out This Form Study it Carefully.

Read and Follow Instructions—Print Plainly in Ink or Use Typewriter. DO NOT Use Pencil—All Signatures Must Be in Ink.

Applicant Must Not Write In Space Below

MAY 1 1950
Date Application Was Received

Batch 16170 Control Number 65288

1—Name of Applicant.

GRIFFITH,   Arthur   Raymond
Last   First   Middle or Initial

2—Address to Which CHECK and MAIL is to be Sent.

1007 SE 15th Avenue   Portland   Multnomah   Oregon
House No. St. R. D. P. O. Box   City or Town   County   State

Active Domestic Service

Months 47 $ 420

Days $

Amount Due $

3—Date and Place of Birth.

Sept. 18, 1921   Altoona   Blair   Penna.
Month Day Year   City or Town   County   State

Active Foreign Service

Months $

Days $

Amount Due $

4—Name Under Which Applicant Served In World War II.

GRIFFITH,   Arthur   Raymond
Last   First   Middle or Initial

5—Date of Beginning and Date of Ending of Each Period of Service Between December 7, 1941 and March 2, 1946 (Both Dates Inclusive) During Which Applicant Was In DOMESTIC SERVICE.

Total Amt. Due $ 420

February 23, 1942   January 17, 1946
Date of Beginning   Date of Ending

Audited By

Service Computed By

6—Date of Beginning and Date of Ending of Each Period of Service Between December 7, 1941 and March 2, 1946 (Both Dates Inclusive) During Which Applicant Was In FOREIGN SERVICE.

Amounts Extended By

Approved For Payment

Date DEC 13 1950

XXXXXXXXXXXXXXX none XXXXXXXXXXXXXXX
Date of Beginning   Date of Ending

For A. G.

For Aud. G.

For S. T.

7—Date and Place Applicant Entered Active Service.

Feb. 23, 1942   Pittsburgh, Penna.
Month Day Year   Place

Application Disapproved

By

8—Service or Serial Numbers Assigned To Applicant.

Service No's. 652 20 31

Serial No's.

9—Date and Place Where Applicant Was Separated From Active Service.

January 17, 1946   Personnel Seperation Center
Month Day Year   Sampson, N.Y.   Place

10—Is Applicant Now Serving In Armed Forces On Active Duty?   Yes _____   No X
If Answer Is YES—Be Sure To Have Certificate Executed And Filed With Application—See Instruction Sheet.

11—Mark "X" Above Name To Indicate Sex And Branch of Service.

X   X
Male   Female   Army   Navy   Marine Corps   Coast Guard   Other—Describe

12—Applicant's Residence At Time of Entry Into Active Service.

552 53rd Street   Altoona   Blair   Penn
House No.   Street   R. D.   P. O. Box   City or Town   County   State

13—Applicant Was Registered Under Selective Service As Follows.

4   Altoona   Blair   Penna.
Draft Board No.   City or Town   County   State

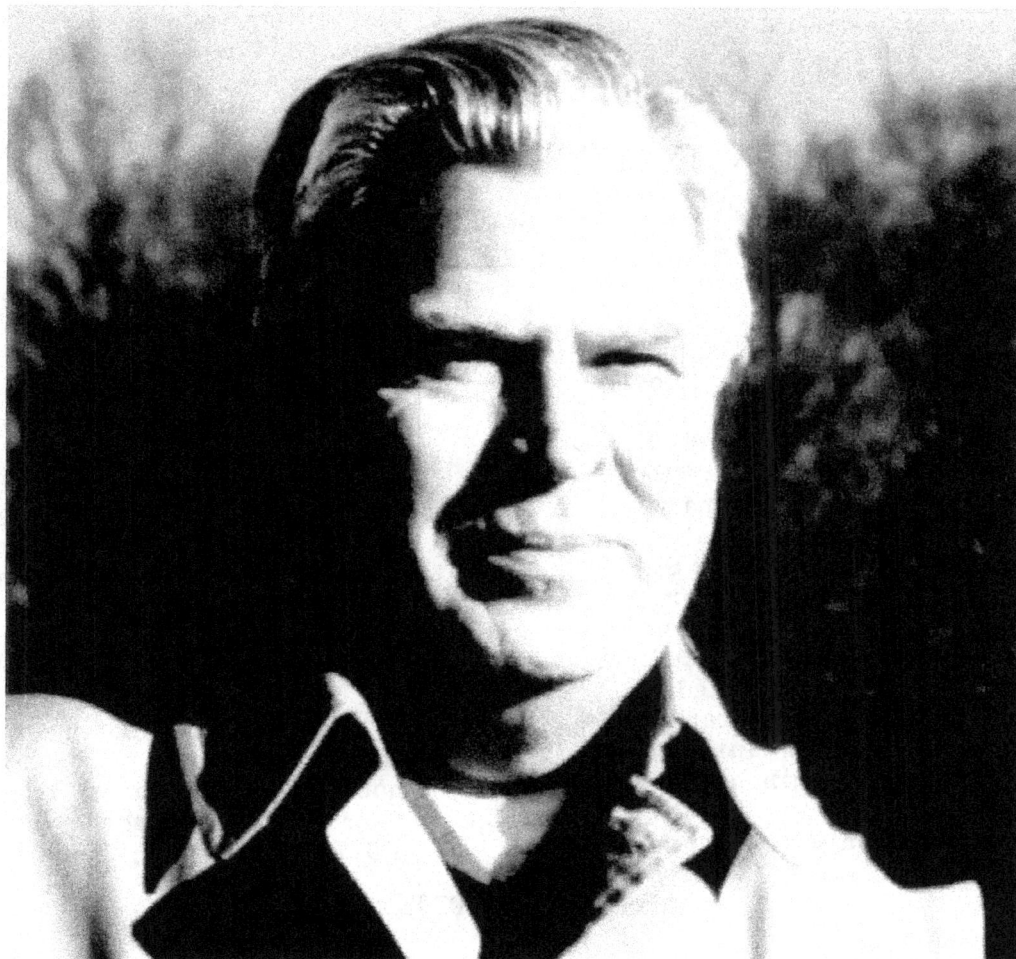

ARTHUR RAYMOND GRIFFITH

E371 JACK RICHARD BRUCKMAN E37

JACK RICHARD BRUCKMAN was born on 18 Aug 1911 in Blair Co., PA and died 10 Jul 1981 in Pinellas Co., FL. He married GERALDINE M. HOOVER in Blair Co., PA, daughter of LISLIE HOOVER and ELMA HESS. She was born in 21 January 1918 in PA and died Oct 1976.

Children of JACK BRUCKMAN and GERALDINE HOOVER are:

    i. THOMAS R. BRUCKMAN (E3711) was born in 1936 in Altoona, Blair Co., PA.

    ii. BEVERLY A. BRUCKMAN (E3712) was born in 1938 in Altoona, Blair Co., PA.

Ref: 50, 42, 12-Ward 14 Altoona Blair Co PA F11, LH Obit Altoona Tribune 03 Dec 1949

Miss Hoover, Jack Bruckman Are Married

Miss Geraldine Hoover, daughter of Mr. and Mrs. Leslie Hoover, 5500 Sixth avenue, and Jack Bruckman, son of Mr. and Mrs. Arthur F. Bruckman, 5810 Beale avenue, were united in marriage on Thanksgiving morning at 10:40 o'clock at Fifty-Eighth Street Methodist church before members of the immediate families and a few intimate friends. Rev. Herbert W. Glassco, pastor, officiated.

The impressive ring ceremony was performed before an altar of palms, ferns, chrysanthemums and pompoms.

Harold Rice, this city, presided at the organ, playing, "O Promise Me," after which Mrs. Glassco sang "I Love You Truly." The bride entered to the strains of the "Wedding March" from Wagner's "Logengrin." The recessional was Mendelssohn's "Wedding March."

The bride was charmingly attired in a royal blue chion velvet gown with hat to match and a short veil. She carried Joanna Hill roses. The brides attendant, Miss Alma Johnston, wore a rust crepe gown with hat to match. She carried yellow and rust chrysanthemums.

John Hoine was the best man. Following the nuptials, dinner was served at the Penn Alto hotel at which the bridal party and the parents of the contracting parties were present.

Mr. Bruckman is associated with his father in business at the A. F. Bruckman Economy store. Mr. and Mrs. Bruckman will be at home to their many friends in their newly furnished apartment, 305 Eighth avenue, Juniata.

Altoona Tribune 02 Dec 1935

E381 RICHARD W. BRUCKMAN E38

RICHARD W. BRUCKMAN was born on 28 May 1920 in Altoona, Blair Co., PA and died 29 Nov 1990 in Baltimore, Baltmore Co., MD. He married VELMA M. CORWIN. She was born on 30 Sep 1909 and died 02 Oct 1999 in Manchester, Carroll Co., MD.

Children of RICHARD BRUCKMAN and VELMA CORWIN are:

i. MERLA AUGUSTA BRUCKMAN (E3811) was born 18 Sep 1927 in MD and died 04 Feb 2011 in Mims, Carroll Co., MD. She married _____ GILCHRIST.

Merla Augusta Gilchrist, 83, of Mims, Fla., died Friday, Feb. 4, 2011. A service will be held at 7 p.m. Thursday at North Brevard Funeral Home in Titusville, Fla.
Carroll County Times 08 Feb 2011

ii. RONALD B. BRUCKMAN (E3812)

Ref: 42

Services for Richard W. Bruckman, a retired accounting officer with the Maryland State Police, will be held at 11 a.m. tomorrow at Eline Funeral Home, 11824 Reisterstown Road. Mr. Bruckman, a resident of Owings Mills, died of an aneurysm Thursday at Sinai Hospital. He was

70. A native of Altoona, Pa., Mr. Bruckman graduated from Altoona High School in 1937. His family later moved to Glen Burnie, and he worked for Eastern Aircraft while attending night school in Baltimore. He retired in 1985 as head accounting officer of the finance division of the Pikesville barracks after 40 years of service and was a member of the Alumni Association. He was also coach of the troopers' basketball team in the mid-1970s. Mr. Bruckman was past president and treasurer of the Reisterstown Lions Club, with 38 years of service, and a member of the Reisterstown Moose Lodge No. 1577 and the Four Seasons Sports Complex in Hampstead. He served on the board of directors of the Baltimore American Savings Bank in Glen Burnie. Mr. Bruckman enjoyed racing his flock of 200 homing pigeons and was a member of the Homing Pigeon Association. He was also active in community work. He is survived by his wife of 46 years, Velma M. Corwin; a daughter, Merla A. Gilchrist of Glen Burnie; a son, Ronald B. Bruckman of Hampstead; two sisters, Eloise Kellenberger and Roselma Felty, both of Glen Burnie; five grandchildren; four great-grandchildren; and one great-great-grandchild. The family has suggested donations be made to the Reisterstown Lions Club, P. O. Box 22, Reisterstown, Md. 21136.

The Baltimore Sun 02 Dec 1990

Richard W. Bruckman, 70, died Nov. 29 at Sinai Hospital in Baltimore. A Baltimore County resident, he was the husband of Velma M. Bruckman. A retired accountant with the Maryland State Police, he also was a board member of the American Savings Bank. In addition to his wife, survivors include a daughter, Merla Gilchrist of Manchester; son, Ronald B. Bruckman of Hampstead; sisters, Eloise Kellenberger and Roselma Felty, both of Anne Arundel County; five grandchildren; four great-grandchildren and one great-great-grandchild.

The Baltimore Sun 09 Dec 1990

E382 ELOISE CLARECE BRUCKMAN E38

ELOISE CLARECE BRUCKMAN was born on 18 Mar 1925 in Altoona, Blair Co., PA. She married PAUL ROSS KELLENBERGER in MD, son of FRANCIS ALBERT KELLENBERGER and HELEN GERTRUDE KNAUFF. He was born on 20 Apr 1925 in MD.

Children of ELOISE BRUCKMAN and PAUL KELLENBERGER are:

  i. CRAIG ALLEN KELLENBERGER (E3821) was born in MD.

  ii. GARY ROSS KELLENBERGER (E3822) was born on 07 Dec 1947 in Baltimore, Baltimore Co., MD and died 02 Apr 1953 in Baltimore, Baltimore Co., MD.

  iii. KAREN MARIE KELLENBERGER (E3823) was born in MD.

Ref: 49

E383 ROSELMA BRUCKMAN E38

ROSELMA BRUCKMAN was born on 03 Jan 1928 in Altoona, Blair Co., PA and died 01 Jan 2010 in Baltimore, Baltimore City Co., MD. She married RICHARD FRANCIS FELTY Sr. He was born on 10 Dec 1925 and died Jan 1986 in Anne Arundel Co., MD. She is buried in Meadowridge Memorial Park, Elkridge, Howard Co., MD.

Children of ROSELMA BRUCKMAN and RICHARD FELTY are:

    i. RICHARD FRANCIS FELTY Jr. (E3831)

    ii. BARRY W. FELTY (E3832)

Ref: 42, 26

Roselma Ruth Felty, 81, a resident of Glen Burnie for 57 years, died of natural causes Jan. 1, 2010. She was born Jan. 3, 1928, in Altoona, Pa. She graduated from Glen Burnie High School. She worked for over 22 years at Corcoran Elementary School until she retired. She had also worked part-time for Ziegler's Florist. Roselma was an active member of the Glen Burnie United Methodist Church where she served as treasurer for the Women's Circle for many years. She also belonged to the Retired Teachers Association. She had a great love of the outdoors, always enjoyed camping in her RV, and was very talented with crafting. She was preceded in death by her husband of 36 years, Richard F. Felty Sr.; and her brother, Richard Bruckman. She is survived by her sons, Richard Jr. of Florida and Barry W. Felty of Glen Burnie; sister, Eloise Kellenberger of Glen Burnie; two grandchildren and nine great-grandchildren. Funeral services will be held at 10 a.m. Wednesday, Jan. 6 at Kirkley-Ruddick Funeral Home, 421 Crain Hwy. S.E. in Glen Burnie. Interment Meadowridge Memorial Park. In lieu of flowers, donations may be made in her name to the Glen Burnie UMC, 2nd Ave. & Crain Hwy. SE, Glen Burnie, MD 21061. For more information or to post condolences, please visit www.kirkleyruddickfuneralhome.com

Maryland Gazette 06 Jan 2010

E412 GEORGE WILLIAM PETRY Sr. E41

GEORGE WILLIAM PETRY Sr. was born in Jun 1896 in Somerset Co., PA and died Sep 1975 in PA. He married MAZIE SHAFFER in Johnstown, Cambria Co., PA. She was born 1931 in PA.

Children of GEORGE PETRY Sr. and MAZIE SHAFFER are:

    i. SANFORD PETRY (E4121) married HAZEL _____.

    ii. EUGENE PETRY (E4122) married VIVIAN _____.

    iii. GEORGE WILLIAM PETRY Jr. (E4123)

    iv. MELROY "MELVIN" PETRY (E4124)

    v. ROBERT PETRY (E4125) married BLANCHE _____.

Ref: 26, 11-Johnstown Cambria Co PA F376, 42, Son Melroy's Obit

E421 FREDERICK W. DELOZIER E42

FREDERICK W. DELOZIER was born in 20 Apr 1900 in Somerset Co., PA and died 27 Oct 1955. He married ELIZABETH LEYDIG, daughter of ISAIAH DANIEL LEYDIG and

ANNA BELLE COLEMAN. She was born on 29 Apr 1900 in Glencoe, Somerset Co., PA and died 21 Apr 1993 in Elyria, Lorain Co. OH. Both are buried in Mt. Lebanon Reformed Church Cemetery, Somerset Co., PA.

Children of FREDERICK DELOZIER and ELIZABETH LEYDIG are:

   i. MARION V. DELOZIER (E4211)

   ii. WILLIAM DELOZIER (E4212) was born in 1936 in Connellsville, Fayette Co., PA.

   iii. ROBERT R. DELOZIER (E4213) was born in 1936 in Connellsville, Fayette Co., PA.

Ref: 44, 12-Clewiston Hendry Co FL F270

Elizabeth L. DeLozier, 92, Elyria, Ohio, formerly of Connellsville, Pa., Baltimore, Md. and Clewiston, Fla., died April 21, 1993, at the home of her daughter. Born April 29, 1900 in Glencoe. Preceded in death by her husband, Fred, in 1955. Survived by daughter, Mrs. Loyal (Marion) Cowan, Elyria, Ohio; and son, William, Fuqua-Varina, N.C.; seven grandchildren and four great-grandchildren. Her father, I.D. Leydig, had owned the general store in Glencoe. She is a 1918 graduate of Meyersdale High School, member of Community United Methodist Church, Elyria, Ohio; and Dorcas Circle of the church; 73-year-member of the Cumberland Chapter Order of the Eastern Star. Family will receive friends from 2-4 and 7-9 p.m. Friday at Deaner Funeral Home, Berlin, where Eastern Star service will be held Friday at 7:30 p.m. Funeral service at 11 a.m. Saturday, with the Rev. W. Stephen Morse officiating. Interment, Mount Lebanon Cemetery.

Daily American 22 Apr 1993

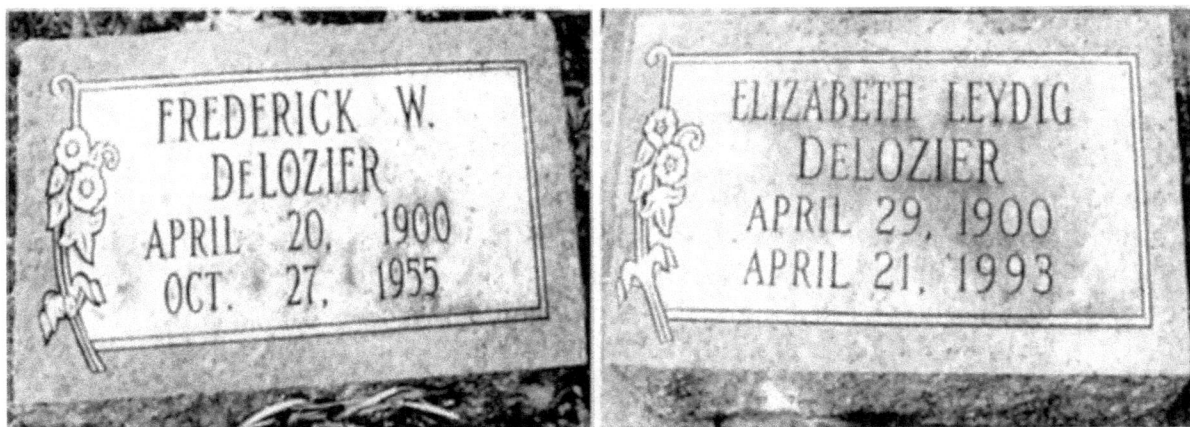

E422 ALMA A. DELOZIER E42

ALMA A. DELOZIER was born on 20 May 1901 in Salisbury, Somerset Co., PA and died 18 Dec 19975 In Somerset, Somerset Co,, PA. She married DEWEY A. SMITH. He died 03 Jul 1962 in Somerset Co., PA.

Children of ALMA DELOZIER and DEWEY SMITH are:

   i. MARIETTA L. SMITH (E4221)

ii. CHESTER A. SMITH (E4222) was born on 09 Sep 1925 in Boswell, Somerset Co., PA and died 06 Feb 2003 in Acosta, Somerset Co., PA. He married ROSE MARIE KOZEL in Somerset Co., PA.

> Chester A. Smith, 77, Acosta, died Feb. 6, 2003 at home. Born Sept. 9, 1925 in Boswell, son of the late Dewey and Alma (DeLozier) Smith. Survived by wife of 53 years, the former Rose Marie Kozel and sisters, Marietta, widow of Milton Griffin, Boswell, Helen, widow of Ray Weigle, Friedens, Roberta Ling-Kaulp, Mansfield, Ohio, and Emma Jean, married to Ray Charlton, Hollidaysburg. Also survived by sister-in-law and brother-in-law, Josephine and Rudy Zanoni, Acosta, and numerous nieces and nephews. Member of the former Boswell High School class of 1944. Navy veteran of World War II having served in the Pacific Theater of Operation. Retired cloth cutter of the former Dorfman and Hoffman Garment Factory, with over 39 years service. A member of All Saints Catholic Parish and the Shanksville American Legion. Former member of the Knights of Columbus. Friends received from 2 to 9 p.m. Friday at the Hoffman Funeral Home, Main Street, Boswell, where vigil for the deceased will be held at 2 p.m. Friday. Funeral Mass at 10 a.m. Saturday at All Saints Chapel, Acosta. The Rev. Father Justin A. Ratajcza OFM Conv. celebrant. Committal Somerset County Memorial Park with graveside military rite in charge of the Somerset County Honor Guard.
>
> Daily American, February 7, 2003

iii. HELEN E. SMITH (E4223)

iv. ROBERTA A. SMITH (E4224) was born in Somerset Co., PA married DONALD C. LING-KAULP in Somerset Co., PA.

v. EMMA JEAN SMITH (E4225)

Ref: 44

Mrs. Alma A. Smith, 74, of 202 Center Street, Boswell, died Dec. 18, 1975, in Somerset Community Hospital. Born May 20, 1901, in Salisbury, she was a daughter of George G. and Emma F. (Petry) Delozier. She was preceded in death by her husband, Dewey A. Smith, July 3, 1962; her parents and two brothers. Surviving are these children: Marietta L., wife of Milton E. Giffin of Boswell; Chester A., married to the former Rose Marie Kozel of Acosta; Helen E., wife of Ray T. Weigle of Friedens RD 2; Roberta A., wife of Donald C. Ling, of Mansfield, Ohio; Emma Jean, wife of Jason R. Charlton of Bridgeville, Del,; also eight grandchildren and three great-grandchildren. She was a sister of Mrs. Mary L. Hartman of Glencoe; Mrs. Emma E. Ludy of Berlin; George A. Delozier, Connellsville; Walter G. and Arthur A., both of Cumberland, Md. An aunt, Mrs. Grace Petry, of Salisbury, also survives. Mrs. Smith was a long-time active member of the Boswell Church of God, where she was the pianist and taught Sunday School for more than 30 years. Funeral service was held Sunday afternoon at Boswell Church of God with the Rev. Samuel E. Charlton and the Rev. David N. Lykens officiating. Interment in Lebanon Cemetery.

Meyersdale Republic 25 Dec 1975

E423 MARY M. DELOZIER E42

MARY M. DELOZIER was born on 15 Feb 1903 in Somerset Co., PA and died 04 Jul 1987 in Somerset, Somerset Co., PA. She married JOHN W. HARTMAN in Somerset Co., PA. He was born on 16 Nov 1901 Allegheny Twp., Somerset Co., PA and died 08 Jul 1980 in Glencoe, Somerset Co., PA.

Children of MARY DELOZIER and JOHN HARTMAN are:

  i. JAMES E. HARTMAN (E4231)

Ref: 44, 11-Northampton Twp Somerset Co PA F78

John W. Hartman, 78, Glencoe, died July 8, 1980, at Jeanette Hospital. He was born Nov. 16, 1901, in Allegheny Township, and was reared by grandparents, the late Annie and Alonzo Hartman. He is survived by his wife, former Mary Delozier; son James E. Hartman, Somerset; grandchildren: David Hartman, Somerset; Dennis Hartman, Washington; and Donna Hartman, Somerset; great-grandchild Wesley Scott, Washington. He was a former employee of B & O Railroad. He was a former member Mt. Lebanon United Church of Christ, where he served as an elder, deacon and trustee. Following the closing of that church he attended Glencoe United Church of Christ. He was a member of the Brotherhood of Maintenance of Way Lodge 1556. Friends were received at the Johnson-Kuhlman Funeral Home, Berlin, where services were held with the Rev. William N. Hay and the Rev. Robert Hoffman officiating. Interment, Mt. Lebanon Cemetery.

The Republic 17 Jul 1980

Mary M. Hartman, 84, Glencoe, died July 4, 1987, at Somerset Community Hospital. Born Feb. 15, 1903, in Salisbury, daughter of George G. and Emma (Petry) DeLozier. Preceded in death by parents; husband, John W.; three brothers and two sisters. Survived by son, James E. of Somerset; and these grandchildren: David, Pittsburgh; Denis, Washington, Pa.; and Donna of Somerset; and three great-grandchildren. Also survived by brother, George A. DeLozier, Connellsville. Member of Glencoe United Church of Christ and Somerset County Historical Society. Friends will be received 7-9 p.m. Monday and 2-4 and 7-9 p.m. Tuesday at the Johnson-Kuhlman Funeral Home where services will be held 11 a.m. Wednesday, the Rev. William N. Hay officiating. Interment, Mt. Lebanon Cemetery.

Daily American 06 Jul 1987

E425 WALTER GERBER DELOZIER E42

WALTER GERBER DELOZIER was born on 22 Apr 1910 in Somerset Co., PA and died 24 Dec 1983 Somerset Co., PA. He married ELIZABETH J. LUDY.

  i. MARY E. DELOZIER (E4251) was born in 1923 in Somerset Co., PA. She married _____ BENSON.

  ii. FREDA M. DELOZIER (E4252) was born in 1925 in Somerset Co., PA. She married _____ BENSON.

iii. JANE DELOZIER (E4253) was born in 1939 in Somerset Co., PA. She married _____ LAFFERTY.

iv. MAXINE J. DELOZIER (E4254)

Ref: 44, 12-Wellersburg Somerset Co PA F79

Walter G. DeLozier, 73, of 625 Elm Street, died December 24, 1983, at Memorial Hospital. Born April 22, 1910 in Somerset County, he was a son of the late George G. and DeLozier and Emma (Petry) Delozier. He was a retired B. and O. Railroad carman helper. He was a member of Kingsley United Methodist Church; the Brotherhood of Railway Carmen of America, and Fort Cumberland Lodge 211, AF&AM. Surviving are his widow, Mrs. Elizabeth J. (Ludy) DeLozier; four daughters, Mrs. Mary Benson, Mrs. Freda Benson and Mrs. Jane Lafferty, all of Cumberland, Maryland; Mrs. Maxine Furedy, Pittsburgh; one brother, George A. DeLozier, Connellsville; one sister, Mrs. Mary Hartman, Glencoe; 16 grandchildren and two great-grandchildren. Friends were received at the Scarpelli Funeral Home. A Masonic memorial service was held Tuesday at 7:30 p.m. Services were conducted at the funeral home Wednesday at 1 p.m. by the Rev. Earl E. Mason. Interment will be in Sunset Memorial Park. Pallbearers, all grandsons, were Michael Benson, Terry G. Benson, George S. Benson, William Benson, Joseph Benson and Albert Furedy. Honorary pallbearers were Walter Benson, Steven Furedy and David Furedy.

The Republican 29 Dec 1983

E426 EMMA E. DELOZIER E42

EMMA E. DELOZIER was born on 21 Sep 1912 in Glencoe, Somerset Co., PA and died 13 Mar 1976 in Johnstown, Cambria Co., PA. She married JAMES E. LUDY in Somerset Co., PA, son of JACOB LUDY and MAUDE DIVELY. He was born on 02 Jul 1910 in Scottdale, Westmoreland Co., PA.

Children of EMMA DELOZIER and JAMES LUDY are:

i. JAMES W. LUDY (E4261) was born in 1934 in Somerset Co., PA.

ii. DALE F. LUDY (E4262)

iii. WAYNE A. LUDY (E4263) was born in Somerset Co., PA. He married BESSIE FOSTER.

iv. MARY L. LUDY (E4264) was born in Somerset Co., PA. She married HOMER KREINBROOK

Ref: 44, 12-Northampton Twp Somerset Co PA F57

Mrs. Emma E. Ludy, 63, of Berlin, died March 13, 1976, in Mercy Hospital, Johnstown. She was born Sept. 21, 1912, in Glencoe, the daughter of the late George G. and Emma (Petry) Delozier. Preceded in death by two brothers and one sister. Survived by her husband, James E., and these children: Wayne A., Greenwood, Ind.; James W., Levittown, Pa.; Dale F., Enon, Ohio; and Mrs. Mary L. Kreinbrook, Berlin; also 13 grandchildren and one great-grandchild. She was a sister of Mrs. John (Mary) Hartman, Glencoe; Albert, Connellsville; Walter G. and Arthur, both of Cumberland, Md. She was a member of Holy Trinity Lutheran Church, Berlin. Friends are being received in the Johnson and Son Funeral Home, Berlin, where services will be held Tuesday at 2 p.m. with the Rev. Gene J. Abel officiating. Interment, Mt. Lebanon Cemetery.

Somerset American 15 Mar 1976

James E. Ludy, 85, Berlin, died Nov. 15, 1995, at Somerset Hospital. Born July 2, 1910, in Scottsdale, son of Jacob and Mary Jane (Todd) Ludy. Preceded in death by parents; stepmother, Maude (Dively) Ludy, his wife, the former Emma DeLozier; brothers: William, Charles, Edwin, Carl and Jacob Benjamin, and a sister, Sarah Smith. Survived by these children: Wayne A. Miller, married to former Bessie Foster of Indianapolis, Ind.; James W. Ludy of Camp Hill, Dale F. Ludy, married to former Janice Robbins of Seminole, Fla., and Mrs. Homer (Mary) Kreinbrook of Berlin. Also 13 grandchildren, 15 great-grandchildren and a special great-granddaughter, Brittany. Brother of Victor G. of Meyersdale; Elizabeth DeLozier, Cumberland, Md.; Anna Leister, Harry and Noah J., all of Glencoe; Frank of Williamsport, Mary Trent of Friedens, Elaine Werner of Annadale, Va.; Darlene K. Shultz of Farrell, and Sandra Nicholson of Gallup, N.M. Retired from former B&O Railroad. Private service at the convenience of the family. Memorial contributions may be given to the American Cancer Society. Arrangements by Deaner Funeral Home, Berlin.

Daily American 17 Nov 1995

E427 ARTHUR AMERICUS DELOZIER E42

ARTHUR AMERICUS DELOZIER was born on 19 Sep 1914 in Glencoe, Somerset Co., PA and died 21 Mar 1983 in Martinsburg, Berkeley Co., WV. He married EVA W. POWNALL, daughter of WILLIAM M. POWNALL and EMMA LOUISE PARSONS. She was born on 21 Sep 1922 in Springfield, Hampshire Co., WV. Both are buried in Rocky Gap Veterans Cemetery, Flintstone, Allegany Co., MD.

Children of ARTHUR DELOZIER and EVA POWNALL are:

    i. ROGER A. DELOZIER (E4271)

    ii. BARRY A. DELOZIER (E4272) He married SUSIE.

    iii. AUDREY MARTZ DELOZIER (E4273) _____ HYNDMAN

    iv. CONNIE DELOZIER (E4274)

    v. SHEILA R. DELOZIER (E4275)

Ref: 44, 26

Arthur A. DeLozier, 68, of 1037 Myrtle Street, Cumberland, Md., died March 21, 1983 at the Veterans Administration Center in Martinsburg, W.Va. He was born Sept 19, 1914 in Glencoe, and was the son of the late George DeLozier and Emma (Petry) DeLozier. He was a retired foreman for the Kelly-Springfield Tire Company and was a veteran of Navy service in World War II and the Korean Conflict. He was a member of Christ United Methodist Church; a member and past member of Fort Cumberland Lodge 211, AF&AM; a member of the Scottish Rite, Ali

Ghan Shrine, Ali Ghan Shrine Band, The Past Masters Unit, the Tall Cedars of Lebanon and a past patron of the Order of the Eastern Star. He was a former manager of the Ali Ghan Hot Stove baseball team and was a former vice president and member of the board of directors of the Hot Stove League. He is survived by his widow, Mrs. Eva W. (Pownall) DeLozier; two sons, Roger A. DeLozier, Cresaptown, Maryland; Barry A. DeLozier, Richmond, Virginia; three daughters, Mrs. Audrey Martz, Hyndman; Mrs. Connie Winebrenner, Hancock, Maryland; Mrs. Sheila R. Densock, Cumberland; two brothers, Albert DeLozier, Connellsville; Walter G. DeLozier, Cumberland; one sister, Mrs. Mary Hartman, Glencoe; 11 grandchildren and two great-grandchildren. Friends were received at the Scarpelli Funeral Home. Fort Cumberland Lodge will conduct a memorial service at the funeral home Wednesday at 7:30 p.m.

The Republic 24 Mar 1983

CUMBERLAND, MD -Eva W. DeLozier, 90, of Cumberland, passed away on Monday, March 25, 2013, at Allegany, Health Nursing and Rehab Center. Born on September 21, 1922, in Springfield, W Va., she was the daughter of the late William M. and Emma Louise (Parsons) Pownall. She was preceded in death by her husband, Arthur A. "Shorty" DeLozier, and a brother, Thomas "Top" Pownall. Eva was a 1941 graduate of Fort Hill High School and a member of Christ United Methodist Church, the Eastern Star Cumberland Chapter #56 and Re Temple Daughters of the Nile. She was a homemaker. Surviving is a daughter, Sheila R. Densock and husband Joe, Cumberland: her son; Barry A. DeLozier and wife Susie, Richmond, Va., grandchildren: Chere A. Conley and husband Matt; Brett J. Densock and wife Michele both of Cumberland; Jeremy DeLozier; Angela DeLozier; Daniel Delozier and Devin DeLozier; eight great-grandchildren; Cory, Brooklyn, Hayden, Sydney, Brayden, Brandon, Alea and Elliot and a sister, Dorothy I. Murphy, Cumberland. Friends will be received at the Scarpelli Funeral Home, P.A., 108 Virginia Ave., Cumberland, (www.scarpellifh.com) on Friday, March 29, 2013 from 11:00 until Noon. A funeral service will be conducted at the funeral home on Friday at Noon with Rev. Wayne Turner officiating. Interment will be in Maryland State Veteran's Cemetery, Rocky Gap.

Scarpelli Funeral Home (www.scarpellifh.com/obits.htm)

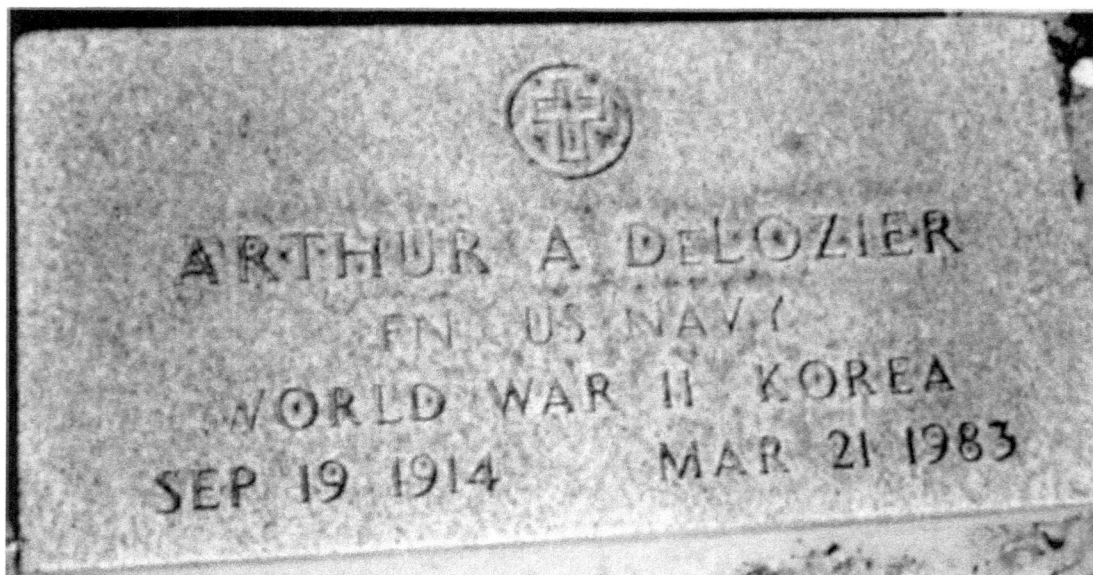

ARTHUR A DELOZIER
FN US NAVY
WORLD WAR II KOREA
SEP 19 1914   MAR 21 1983

Form No. 1 ⬦⬦⬦-10

APPLICATION FOR WORLD WAR II COMPENSATION—TO BE USED BY HONORABLY DISCHARGED VETERAN OR PERSON STILL IN SERVICE

IMPORTANT—Before Filling Out This Form Study it Carefully.

Read and Follow Instructions—Print Plainly in Ink or Use Typewriter. DO NOT Use Pencil—All Signatures Must Be in Ink.

Applicant Must Not Write In Space Below

1—Name of Applicant.

Delozier Arthur A.

Last   First   Middle or Initial

MAY 6 1950
Date Application Was Received

Batch Control Number

17463   62794

2—Address to Which CHECK and MAIL is to be Sent.

625 Elm St.   Cumberland, Allegany   Md.

House No, St. R. D. P. O. Box   City or Town   County   State

Active Domestic Service

Months	$	
Days	5	$
Amount Due	$	50

3—Date and Place of Birth.

9/19/14 Glencoe Pa

Month   Day   Year   City or Town   County   State

Active Foreign Service

Months	$	
Days	$	
Amount Due	$	

4—Name Under Which Applicant Served In World War II.

same

Last   First   Middle or Initial

Total Amt. Due $ 50

5—Date of Beginning and Date of Ending of Each Period of Service Between December 7, 1941 and March 2, 1946 (Both Dates Inclusive) During Which Applicant Was In DOMESTIC SERVICE.

5/4/45   4 – 42   10/14/45

Date of Beginning   Date of Ending

Audited By

Service Computed By

6—Date of Beginning and Date of Ending of Each Period of Service Between December 7, 1941 and March 2, 1946 (Both Dates Inclusive) During Which Applicant Was In FOREIGN SERVICE.

None

Date of Beginning   Date of Ending

Amounts Extended By

Approved For Payment

Date   JUN 30 1950

For A. G.

For Aud. G.

For S. T.

7—Date and Place Applicant Entered Active Service.

5/4/45   Altoona Pa

Month   Day   Year   Place

Application Disapproved

By

8—Service or Serial Numbers Assigned To Applicant.

Service No's.   985 95 69

Serial No's.

9—Date and Place Where Applicant Was Separated From Active Service.

10/14/45   Bainbrige Md   660 553

Month   Day   Year   Place

10—Is Applicant Now Serving In Armed Forces On Active Duty?   Yes _____   No X

If Answer Is YES—Be Sure To Have Certificate Executed And Filed With Application—See Instruction Sheet.

11—Mark "X" Above Name To Indicate Sex And Branch of Service.

X   X

Male   Female   Army   Navy   Marine Corps   Coast Guard   Other—Describe

12—Applicant's Residence At Time of Entry Into Active Service.

Hyndman Pa

House No.   Street   R. D.   P. O. Box   City or Town   County   State

13—Applicant Was Registered Under Selective Service As Follows.

3   Bedford   Bedford   Pa

Draft Board No.   City or Town   County   State

E431 VESTA F. SHARP E43

VESTA F. SHARP was born in 1903 in Somerset Co., PA. She married GILLESPIE B. RHODES on 05 Nov 1921 in Elk Lick Twp., Somerset Co., PA, son of SAMUEL D. RHODES and MARIA MORGRET.

Children of VESTA SHARP and GILLESPIE RHODES are:

i. LOIS MAE RHODES (E4311) married (1) GEORGE A. DAYOOB. She married (2) FRED BENDER.

ii. DELORES J. RHODES (E4312) married DOYAL ABBOTT.

iii. GERALD B. RHODES (E4313)

Ref: 44, 54, 11-Larimer Somerset Co PA F99

E432 ANNIE J. SHARP E43

ANNIE J. SHARP was born on 28 Dec 1903 in Salisbury, Somerset Co., PA and died 24 Oct 1986 in Baden, Beaver Co., PA. She married CHARLES F. HENRY in Somerset Co., PA. He was born 12 Aug 1899 in Hancock, Washington Co., MD and died 26 Aug 1983 in Meyersdale, Somerset Co., PA, son of ORRICK L. HENRY and SUSAN DIBELBLISS. Both are buried in Union Cemetery, Meyersdale, Somerset Co., PA.

Children of ANNIE SHARP and CHARLES HENRY are:

i. JACK A. HENRY (E4321)

ii. HAROLD H. HENRY was born on 07 May 1926 in Meyersdale, Somerset Co., PA and died 24 Sep 2007 in Central City, Somerset Co., PA. He married MARILYN PYATT in Somerset Co., PA, daughter of RICHARD PYATT and RUTH BERKDALE.

Harold H. Henry, 81, Central City, died Sept. 24, 2007, at Select Specialty Hospital. Born May 7, 1926, in Meyersdale, the son of Charles F. and Anna (Sharp) Henry. Preceded in death by parents and a brother, Jack. Survived by wife, the former Marilyn Pyatt; dear in-laws, Richard and Ruth Berkebile, Central City; Dale and Carol Mowry, Berlin; Paul and Barbara Albright, Garrett; Maxine Lehman, Berlin; Robert and Marietta Sicheri, Frostburg, Md.; and Lawrence and Shirley Sicheri, Ridgely, W.Va.; and also survived by numerous nieces and nephews. Harold was a retired surveyor and a U.S. Navy veteran of World War II. A member of the Central City VFW and American Posts as well as various other organizations. An avid gardener, who enjoyed sharing his produce with family and friends. Friends will be received from 4 to 8 p.m. Wednesday at the Mulcahy Funeral Home, where service will be held 11 a.m. Thursday. The Rev. John Jackson officiating. Committal Union Cemetery, Meyersdale. Graveside military rites by VFW Post 554.
Daily American 26 Sep 2007

Ref: 44, 12-Ward 3 Meyersdale Somerset Co PA F72

Charles F. Henry, 84, of Meyersdale died August 26, 1983, Meyersdale Community Hospital. He was born August 12, 1899, in Hancock, Md., a son of the late Orrick L. and Susan (Dibelbliss) Henry. He is survived by his wife, the former Anna J. Sharp; and two sons: Jack A. of Keyser, W.Va.; and Harold H. of Aliquippa; also three grandchildren; and four great-grandchildren. He was the brother of James, of Los Angeles, Calif.; Mrs. Buelah Peebles, Akron, Ohio; and Mrs. Dorothy Long, Meyersdale RD 4. He was a veteran of World War I. He retired from B&O

Railroad as a track foreman after 43 years of service. He was a member of American Legion Post 112 and VFW Post 4503. Friends were received at the Price Funeral Home, Meyersdale, where services were conducted with the Rev. Lloyd Wilson officiating. Interment, Union Cemetery.

The Republic, September 1, 1983

Anna J. Henry, 82, of Meyersdale, died Oct. 24, 1986, in Baden. Born Dec. 28, 1903, in Salisbury, daughter of the late Allen and Lucy (Delozier) Sharp. Also preceded in death by her husband, Charles F. She is survived by a son, Harold H., of Aliquippa; four grandchildren; and four great-grandchildren; two sisters: Mrs. Blanche Tepsich, Youngstown, Ohio; and Mrs. Vesta Rhodes of California. Friends will be received 2-4 and 7-9 p.m. Saturday at the Price Funeral Home, Meyersdale, where services will be conducted at 2 p.m. Sunday, the Rev. Lloyd Wilson officiating. Interment, Union Cemetery, Meyersdale.

Daily American, October 25, 1986

E433 BLANCHE EVELYN SHARP E43

BLANCHE EVELYN SHARP was born on 06 Mar 1907 in Youngstown, Mahoning Co., OH and died 27 Jul 2000 in Youngstown, Mahoning Co., OH. She married (1) CLYDE S. HOUSEL on 02 Feb 1923 in Somerset Co., PA, son of HARVEY ALLEN HOUSEL and ALICE ELIZABETH HOCHSTETLER. He was born on 22 Jul 1901 in Meyersdale, Somerset Co., and died 10 Sep 1970 in Youngstown, Mahoning Co., OH. She married (2) _____ TEPSICH in OH. She and 1st husband are buried in Hochstetler Cemetery, Greenville Twp., Somerset Co., PA.

Children of BLANCHE SHARP and CLYDE HOUSEL are:

　i. CLYDE IRVIN HOUSEL (E4331)

Ref: 44, 12-Ward 2 Meyersdale Somerset Co PA F97, 26, 42, 59

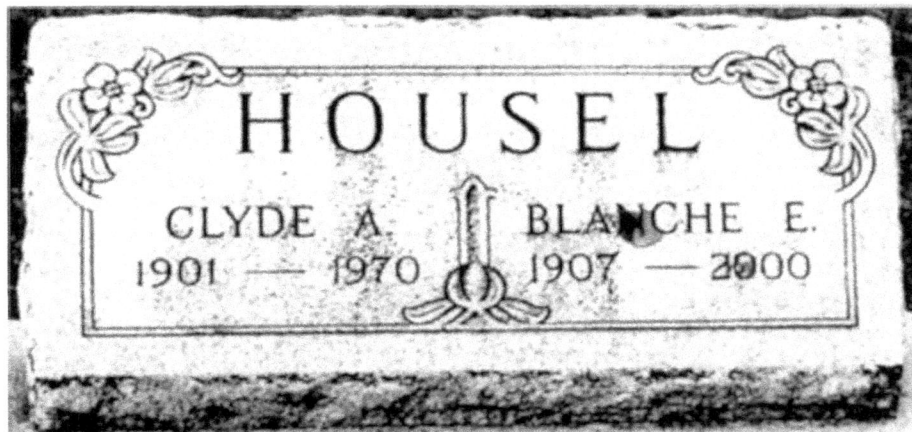

E472 MARGARET DELOZIER E47

MARGARET DELOZIER was born in 1914 in Somerset Co., PA. She married THEODORE SHAW. He was born in 1908 in NY.

Children of MARGARET DELOZIER and THEODORE SHAW are:

   i. BARBARA SHAW (E4721)

   ii. PATRICIA SHAW (E4722)

Ref: 44, 12-North Hempstead Town Nassau Co NY F369

E475 JAMES CHARLES DELOZIER E47

JAMES CHARLES DELOZIER was born on 14 Jun 1918 in PA and died 23 Oct 1977 in Alameda, Alameda Co., CA. He married NORENE JOYCE MORAN on 26 Apr 1943 in Allegheny Co., PA, daughter of THOMAS MORAN and MARY JOYCE. She was born on 29 Dec 1921 in PA and died 01 Oct 1986 in Alameda, Alameda Co., CA. He is buried in Willamette National Cemetery, Portland, Multnomah Co., OR.

Child of JAMES DELOZIER and NORENE MORAN is:

   i. JERRY CHARLES DELOZIER was born on 08 May 1954 in Montgomery, Fayette Co., WV. He married BOBBI JAYNE on 29 Feb 1980 in Alameda, Alameda Co., CA. She was born in 1960. They were divorced on 15 Nov 1982 in Alameda, Alameda Co., CA.

Ref: 33, 42, 54, 76, 77, 78

E481 RUTH J. MULL E48

RUTH J. MULL was born on 10 May 1906 in Somerset Co., PA and died 05 Nov 1954 in Wyandotte, Wayne Co., MI. She married EDISON LANDIS in Somerset Co., PA. He was born in 09 Feb 1901 in PA and died in Apr 1965 in MI.

Children of RUTH MULL and EDISON LANDIS are:

   i. SHIRLEY I. LANDIS (E4811) was born in 1929 in PA.

   ii. HAZEL ARLENE LANDIS (E4812) was born in 04 Aug 1931 in PA and died in 28 Nov 2009 in PA. She married_____ TARPLEY.

   iii. EDISON LANDIS (E4813) was born in 1937 in Wayne Co., MI.

Ref: 12-Tract 806 Encorse Wayne Co MI F19, 43, 42

E482 PETER HOWARD MULL E48

PETER HOWARD MULL was born on 25 Aug 1907 in Sand Patch, Somerset Co., PA and died 14 Jan 1985 Somerset, Somerset Co., PA. He married WILMA EVELYN LESLIE, daughter of RAYMOND MILTON LESLIE and LILLIAN KEISTER. She was born 30 Dec 1913 in Fort Hill, Somerset Co., PA and died 12 Feb 1999 in Somerset, Somerset Co., PA.

   i. LESLIE H. MULL (E4821)

Ref: 12-Somerset Twp Somerset Co PA F574, 44

Peter H. Mull, 77, of Somerset RD 7, died Jan. 14, 1985, at Somerset Community Hospital. Born Aug. 25, 1907, in Sand Patch, son of the late Harvey and Alice (Delozier) Mull. Survived by widow, the former Wilma E. Leslie; a son Leslie, Fort Ashby, W.Va.; and these grandchildren: Leslie H., Eric A. and Rhonda Michelle. He was a brother of: Mrs. Hazel Shaulis, Somerset RD 1; Harvey, Listie; John and Mrs. Carmel (Nora) Perigo, both of Stoystown; and Mrs. John (Dorothy) Dively, Friedens RD 1. He was a retired Penn DOT employee. Friends will be received from 2-4 and 7-9 p.m. Wednesday at the Richard E. Hauger Funeral Home where service will be conducted at 1:30 p.m. Thursday with the Rev. Larry Weigle officiating. Interment, Somerset County Memorial Park.
Daily American 15 Jan 1985

Wilma Evelyn Mull, 85, Somerset, died Feb. 12, 1999, at Somerset Hospital. Born Dec. 30, 1913, in Fort Hill. Daughter of the late Raymond Milton and Lillian (Keister) Leslie. Also preceded in death by husband, Peter Howard Mull, on Jan. 14, 1985, and brother Weldon Leslie. Survived by son, Leslie H. Mull of Fort Ashby, W.Va.; 3 grandchildren: Leslie H. Mull II of Cumberland, Md.; Eric A. Mull of Fort Ashby, and Mrs. Rick (Rhonda) Daddio of Seminole, Fla.; also 8 great-grandchildren: Travis, Garrett, Austin, Ian and Nolan Mull and Ricky, Ryann and Rylee Daddio. A 1932 graduate of Somerset High School. Attended Somerset Alliance Church. Friends received from 2 to 4 and 7 to 9 p.m. Sunday at Hauger-Zeigler Funeral Home, where services will be conducted at 10 a.m. Monday, with the Rev. Walter L. Frankenberry officiating. Interment, Somerset County Memorial Park. Contributions may be made to Somerset Blind Association, 748 S. Center Ave., Somerset, PA 15501.
Daily American 13 Feb 1999

E483 HAZEL ALICE MULL E48

HAZEL ALICE MULL was born on 19 Dec 1908 in Sand Patch, Somerset Co., PA and died 02 May 1995 in Somerset, Somerset Co., PA. She married EARL SHAULIS in Somerset Co., PA, son of ALBERT MARSHALL SHAULIS and ANNA BOWMAN. He was born 21 Oct 1910 in Berlin, Somerset Co., PA and died 17 Jan 1981 in Avon Park, Somerset Co., PA. They were divorced and he married a 2nd time.

Children of HAZEL MULL and EARL SHAULIS are:

i. DOLORES R. SHAULIS (E4831) was born in 1932 in Somerset Co., PA. She married CHARLES A. MILLER.

ii. E. WAYNE SHAULIS (E4832) was born in 1937 in Somerset Co., PA. He married SHIRLEY MOWRY.

iii. ALICE ANN SHAULIS (E4833) was born in 1940 in Somerset Co., PA. She married DAVID O. RAINEY

iv. DOUGLAS A. SHAULIS (E4834) was born in Somerset Co., PA. He married JUDY BARRON

v. LINDA SHAULIS (E4835) was born in Somerset Co., PA. She married ROBERT J. RHODES Jr.

Ref: 12-Somerset Twp Somerset Co PA F215, 44

Earl Shaulis, 70, Box 1112A, Avon Park RD 1, Fla., 33825, died Jan.17, 1981, at home. He was born Oct. 21, 1910, in Berlin, son of the late Albert Marshall and Anna (Bowman) Shaulis. Also preceded in death by an infant sister, Louella. He is survived by his wife, the former Genevieve Bowman; and these children: Dolores (Mrs. Charles A. Miller), Somerset RD 2; E. Wayne, of Rockwood RD 1; Alice (Mrs. David Rainey), Oklawaha, Fla.; Douglas A., Somerset RD 7; and a stepdaughter Cecile (Mrs. Galen Flick), Somerset RD 8; 16 grandchildren and three great-grandchildren. Also survived by two sisters: Mrs. Edna Haugher, Somerset; and Alma (Mrs. Robert O. Barkman), Baltimore, Md. He was a former resident of Somerset and Bedford (Friend's Cove). He was a retired employee of Agway Inc. Memorial services were held at Resurrection Lutheran Church, Avon Park, Fla. In lieu of flowers, please make contributions to the Resurrection Lutheran Church Memorial Fund.
The Republic 22 Jan 1981

Hazel Alice (Mull-Beachley) Shaulis, 86, Friedens RD 2 died May 20, 1995 at Somerset Hospital. Born Dec. 19, 1908 in Sand Patch, Larimer Township. Daughter of the late Harvey L. and Alice R. (Delozier) Mull. Also preceded in death by: foster parents Frank and Anna (Brant) Beachley; sister Ruth Landis; brothers, Peter Mull and Fay Mull and half brother John Mull and foster brother Devon "Barney" Beachley. Survived by these children: Mrs. Charles A. (Dolores) Miller of Somerset RD 2, E. Wayne Shaulis, married to the former Shirley Mowry of Rockwood RD 1, Mrs. David O. (Alice) Rainey of Ocklawaha, Fla.; Douglas A. Shaulis, married to the former Judy Barron of Somerset; Mrs. Robert J. (Linda) Rhodes Jr. of Friedens RD 2. Also 12 grandchildren and 7 great grandchildren. Half sister of Harvey C. Mull, Listie; Mrs. Carmel (Nora) Perigo of Stoystown; Mrs. John F. (Dorothy) Dively of Friedens RD 1 and foster sister Mrs. Jack (Emily) Williams, Cumberland, Md. Lifetime member of the Brethren Church. Retired in 1971 as a cook at Maple Mountain Manor. Friends will be received from 2 to 4 and 7 to 9 p.m. Monday at the Hauger-Zeigler Funeral Home, Somerset, where services will be conducted at 10 a.m. Tuesday, Rev. Sherman H. Berkey and Rev. Ronald D. Beachley officiating. Interment, Somerset County Memorial Park.
Daily American 22 May 1995

E484 SIDNEY FAY MULL E48

SIDNEY FAY MULL was born in 1915 in Somerset Co., PA and died 18 Jul 1970 in Somerset Co., PA. He married FLORENCE MAXINE MENHORN, daughter ELMER GEORGE MENHORN and EMMA ENGLE. She was born on 27 Nov 1918 in Elk Lick, Somerset Co., PA and died 02 Sep 1995 in Myersdale, Somerset Co., PA. Both are buried in Union Cemetery, Meyersdale, Somerset Co., PA.

i. ALLEN WAYNE MULL (E4841)

ii. DONALD RAYMOND MULL (E4842) He married MARY LEE MAYER.

iii. SIDNEY GEORGE MULL (E4843)

iv. JOYCE EILEEN MULL (E4844) married _____ MCGHEE

v. BRENDA KAY MULL (E4845) married FREEMAN HANING.

Ref: 26, 44,

Florence Maxine Mull, 76, of 113 N. Grant St., Apt. 208, Salisbury, died Sept. 2, 1995, at Meyersdale Medical Center. Born Nov. 27, 1918, at Elk Lick, a daughter of the late Elmer George and Emma (Engle) Menhorn. Preceded in death by her husband, Sidney Fay Mull, July 18, 1970; a son, Allen W. Mull, and 2 grandsons, Donald Lee Mull and David Mull. Survived by 2 sons, Donald R. Mull and Sidney G. Mull, both of Salisbury; 2 daughters, Joyce M. McGhee, West Milton, Ohio, and Brenda K. Haning, Salisbury; 2 brothers, George Menhorn, Hayward, Calif., and Dalton Menhorn, Armbrust; 3 sisters: Anna Fike, Meyersdale; Miriam Gray, Trafford, and Frances Ruffner, Youngwood; also 16 grandchildren and 14 great-grandchildren. Member of St. John's United Church of Christ, Salisbury. Retired trimmer for Meyersdale Manufacturing Co. Friends received from 2 to 4 and 7 to 9 p.m. Monday and Tuesday at Newman Funeral Home, Inc., Salisbury. Services will be conducted at 2 p.m. Wednesday at St. John's United Church of Christ, with the Rev. Raymond Brown officiating. Interment, Union Cemetery, Meyersdale. Expressions of sympathy may be directed to St. John's United Church of Christ.

Daily American 05 Sep 1995

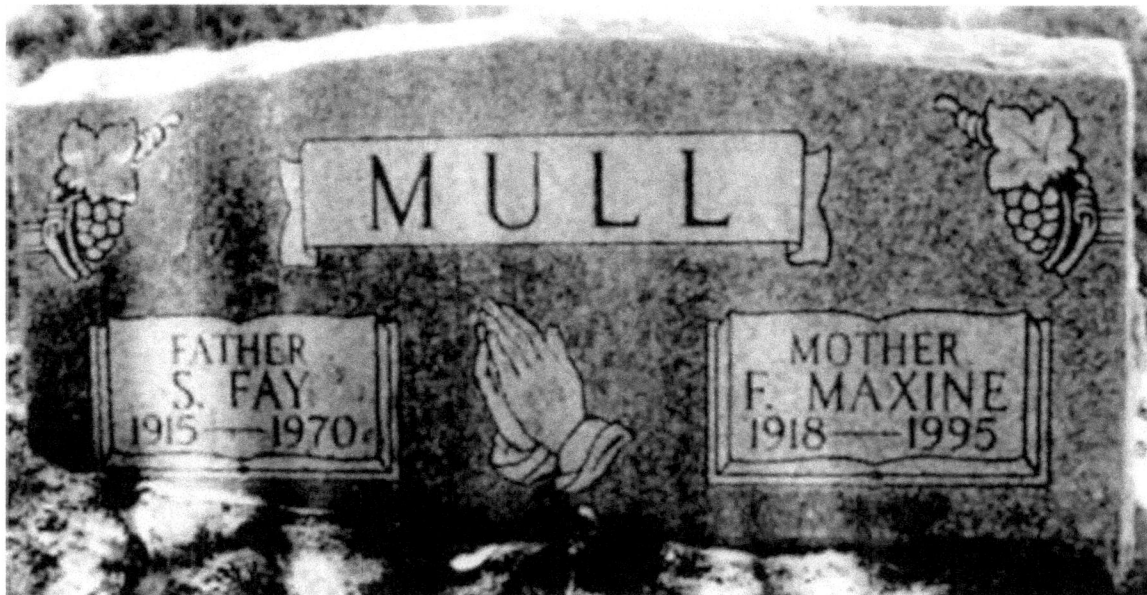

E492 IDA J. SCHROCK E49

IDA J. SCHROCK was born 1914 in Johnstown, Cambria Co., PA. She married PHILLIP A. REESE in Johnstown, Cambria Co., PA. He was born in 1905 in PA.

Child of IDA SCHROCK and PHILLIP REESE is:

i. VIVIAN REESE (E4921) was born in 1937 in Cambria Co., PA.

E3211 RALPH BRYCE MEANS E321

RALPH BRYCE MEANS was born in 10 Mar 1928 in Monroe Twp., Bedford Co., PA and died 16 Oct 2014 in Everett, Bedford Co., PA. He married AUDRA MAXINE WRIGHT on 20 Jun 1952 in Winchester, Frederick Co., VA. He is buried in Old Frame Church Cemetery, Clearville, Bedford Co., PA.

Children of RALPH MEANS and AUDRA WRIGHT are:

   i. DEBRA SUE MEANS (E32111) married _____ SHEFFIELD.

   ii. LYNN BRYCE MEANS (E32112) married SHARON LEE _____.

Ref: 42

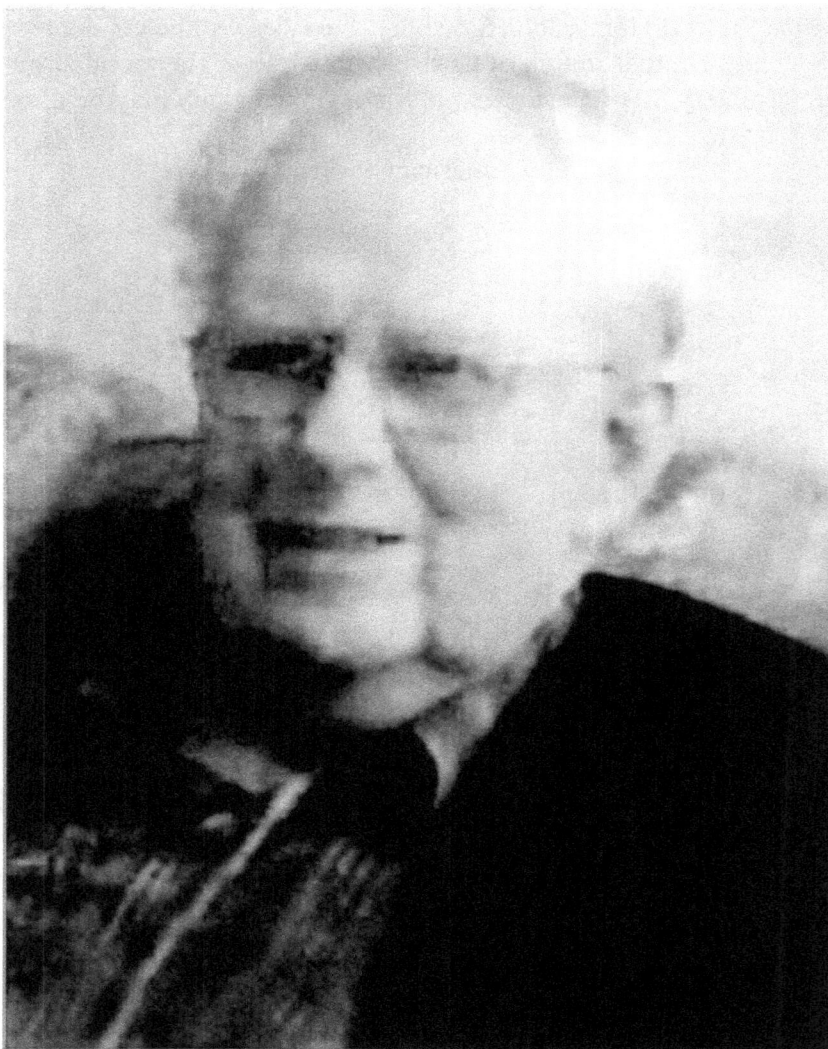

RALPH BRYCE MEANS

Ralph Bryce Means, 86, of Everett, passed away on Thursday, October 16th, 2014 at Donahoe Manor. He was born Saturday, March 10th, 1928 at his family home in Monroe Township, a son of the late Ivan B. Means and Virginia (Weimer) Means. On June 20th, 1952 in Winchester, Virginia, he married Audra Maxine (Wright) Means, who survives along with their daughter Debra Sue Sheffield of Annandale, Virginia, and a son Lynn Bryce Means and wife Sharon Lee Means, of Caswell Beach, North Carolina. Five sisters, Doris Mueller of Lutherville, Maryland Lois Hoagland of Bedford Ruth Borror of York Gail Badaracco and husband Joseph Badaracco of Parkton, Maryland Joyce Pepple and husband J. William Pepple of Everett and many loving nieces, nephews and their families. In addition to his parents, he was preceded in passing away by an infant brother Blair Means. Mr. Means was a faithful member of the Black Valley Federated Church of the Brethren and Christian where he served as the Sunday School Superintendent and Deacon for many years. He also served as an elected official of the Church Board and as a Moderator and Board Chair of the Executive Committee. He was a graduate of Everett High School, Class of 1945, and in 1951, enlisted in the United States Army, serving as a Staff Sergeant with the 23rd Infantry Battalion during the Korean War, earning the Korean Service Medal with one Bronze Service Star, the Combat Infantry Badge, and the United Nations Medal. After his service to our country, Bryce was a member of the Everett American Legion Post #8. For over 35 years, he worked as a Supply Clerk at the Everett Fare Collection Office for the Pennsylvania Turnpike Commission until retiring in 1991, and enjoyed raising Black Angus cattle, hunting deer and turkey, and was an avid Pittsburgh Pirates and Steelers fan who will be greatly missed by his family, friends and community. Funeral services will be held Monday, October 20, 2014 at 11:00am at the Black Valley Federated Church of the Brethren and Christian with Rev. Frank Wheeland officiating. Friends may call at Dalla Valle Funeral Service, Main Street, Everett, on Sunday from 4:00 to 8:00 pm, at the Church on Monday from 10:00 am until the hour of service and share memories online at www.dallavalle-everett.com. Burial will be held at Frame Church Cemetery. Military graveside honors will be conducted by the Everett Honor Guard. Memorial contributions may be made in memory of Bryce to the Black Valley Federated Church, in care of Jack Barney, 145 Shady Maple Lane, Everett, PA 15537 or to Raystown Ambulance Service, 4 South Street, Everett, PA 15537.

Fulton County News 23 Oct 2014

E3215 FLORA GAIL MEANS E321

FLORA GAIL MEANS was born on 04 Nov 1940 in Bedford Co., PA. She married JOSEPH BADARACCO. He was born on 15 Sep 1938.

i. KAREN M. BADARACCO (E32151) was born on 10 Nov 1964 in MD.

Ref: 49

E3511 ESTHER MAY BRUCKMAN E351

ESTHER MAY BRUCKMAN was born on 31 Dec 1953 in Altoona, Blair Co., PA. She married CHARLES DUANE BROOKS on 27 Jul 1974 in Altoona, Blair Co., PA, son of PETER VERNON BROOKS and ANNA LOUISE KINSEL. He was born on 14 Mar 1952 in Crato, Ceara, Brazil.

Children of ESTHER BRUCKMAN and CHARLES BROOKS are:

i. REBECCA ANN BROOKS (E35111) was born 15 May 1975 in Altoona, Blair Co., PA.

ii. RACHEL LOUISE BROOKS (E35112) was born 25 May 1978 in Altoona, Blair Co., PA.

iii. RUTH AMBER BROOKS (E35113) was born 19 May 1986 in Altoona, Blair Co., PA.

Ref: 23-Esther May (Bruckman) Brooks

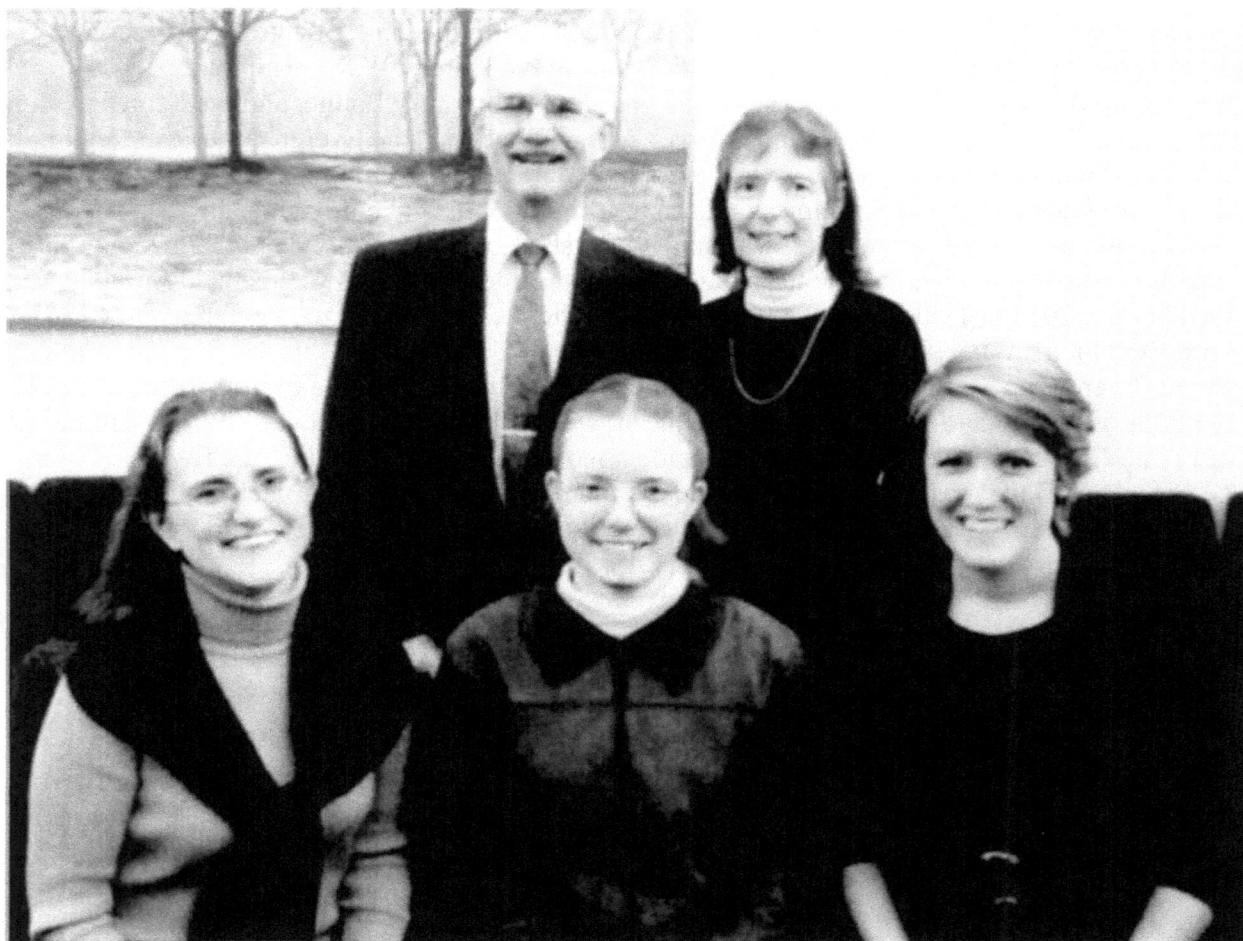

CHARLES DUANE BROOKS and ESTHER MAY (BRUCKMAN) BROOKS
REBECCA BROOKS, RACHEL BROOKS and RUTH BROOKS

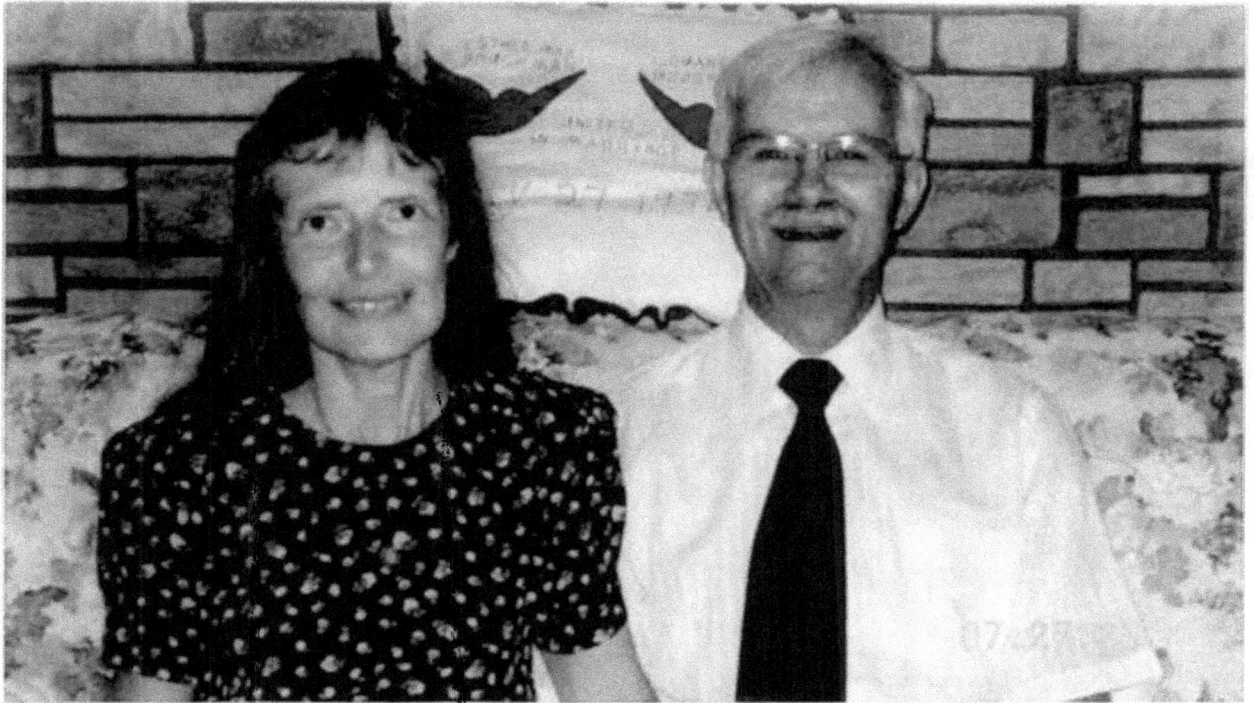

CHARLES DUANE BROOKS and ESTHER MAY (BRUCKMAN) BROOKS

E3531 GERALD THOMAS BRUCKMAN E353

GERALD "JERRY" THOMAS BRUCKMAN was born on 10 Nov 1945. He married (1) LYNDA SMITH WARD, daughter of BUFORD WARD, divorced 26 Jun 1985 in Shelby Co., TN. She was born in 12 Dec 1952 and died 28 Jun 2011 Southaven, De Soto Co., MS. He married (2) CASSANDRA JOY STREET on 28 Apr 1986 in Shelby Co., TN, daughter of HAROLD WAYNE STREET and NELDA RUTH _____. She was born on 26 Sep 1961 in TN.

Children of GERALD BRUCKMAN and LYNDA WARD are:

   i. TERRY RAYMOND BRUCKMAN (E35311)

   ii. MISTI LANE BRUCKMAN (E35312)

   iii. WENDI LYNN BRUCKMAN (E35313)

Children of GERALD BRUCKMAN and CASSANDRA STREET are:

   iv. KRISTY LEE BRUCKMAN (E35314)

Ref: 49, 23-Raymond Clyde Lantz, 23-Wendi Lynn Bruckman

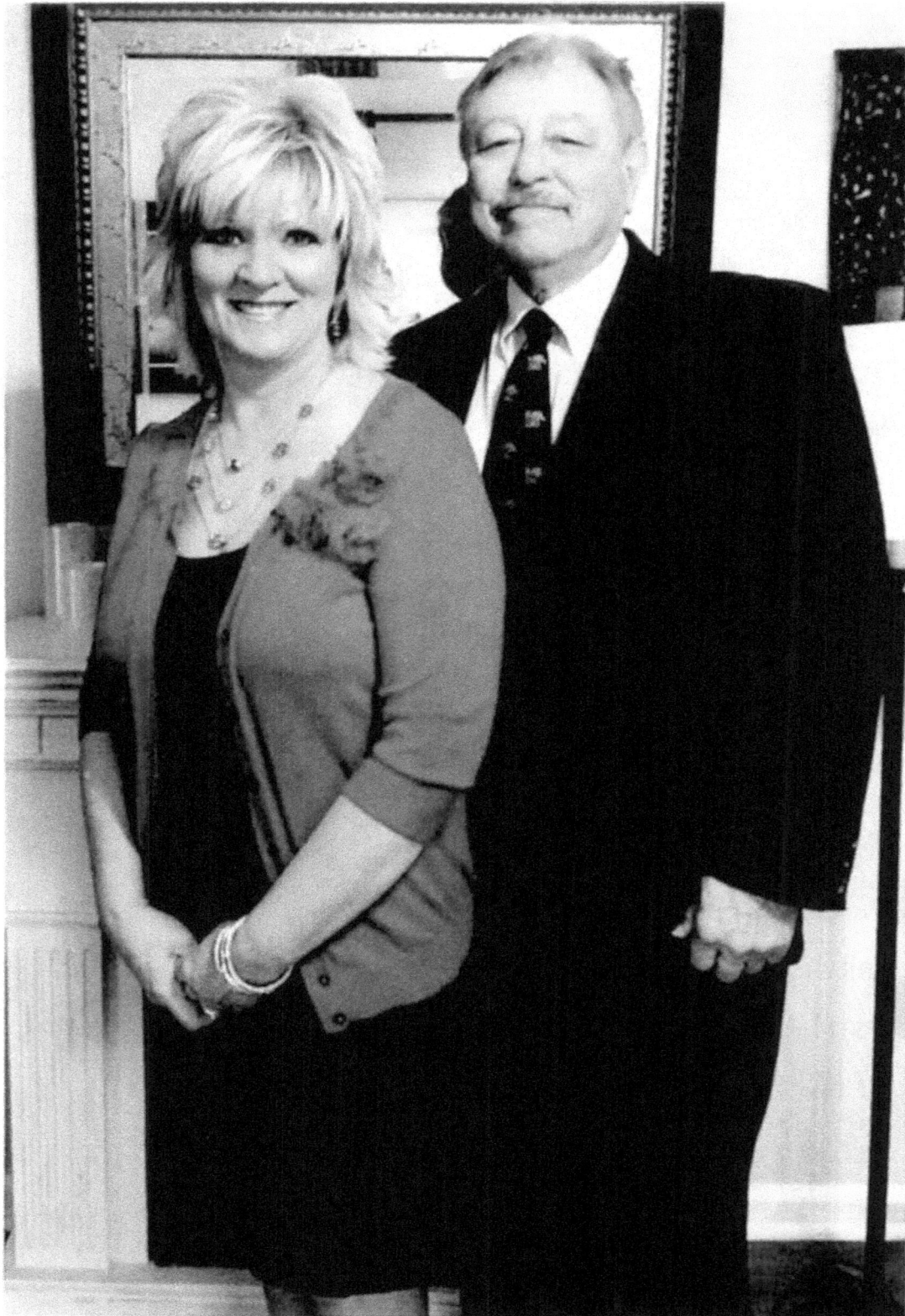

GERALD THOMAS and CASSANDRA JOY (STREET) BRUCKMAN

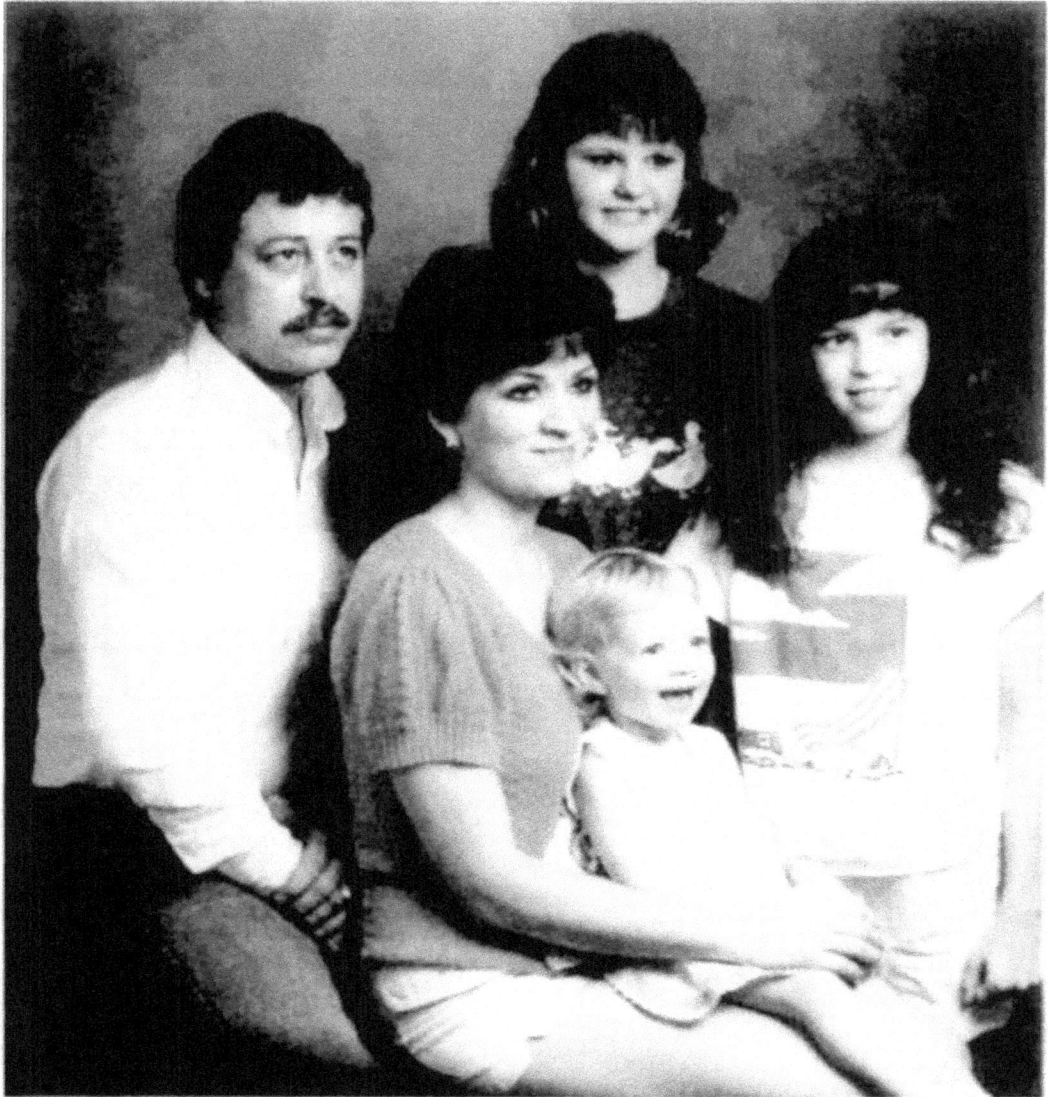

GERALD THOMAS BRUCKMAN, CASSANDRA JOY (STREET) BRUCKMAN, MISTI
LANE BRUCKMAN, WENDI LYNN BRUCKMAN, and MINDY DAWN MILLER
(DAUGHTER OF CASSANDRA STREET and STEPDAUGHTER OF JERRY BRUCKMAN).

E3532 RANDALL EUGENE BRUCKMAN E353

RANDALL "RANDY" EUGENE BRUCKMAN was born on 06 Feb 1957 in Memphis,
Shelby Co., TN. He married PAMELA DENISE BAILEY on 04 Aug 1978 in Memphis, Shelby
Co., TN, daughter of JOHN ALVA BAILEY and DONNA TATE. She was born 30 Dec 1960.

Children of RANDALL BRUCKMAN and PAMELA BAILEY are:

   i. JAMIE LOUISE BRUCKMAN (E35321)

   ii. BAILEY ANN BRUCKMAN (E35322)

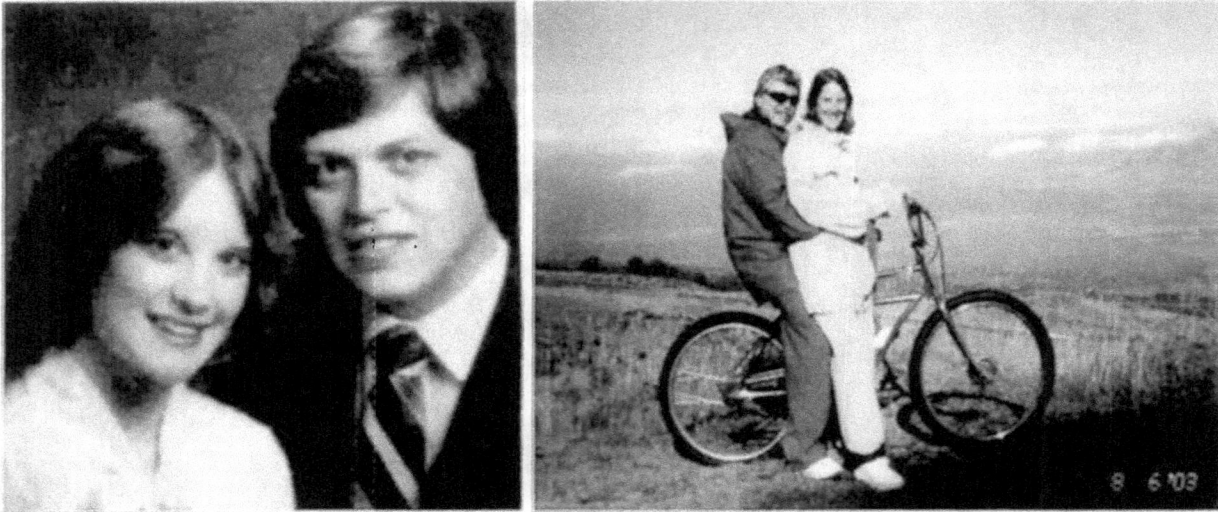

RANDALL EUGENE BRUCKMAN and PAMELA DENISE (BAILEY) BRUCKMAN

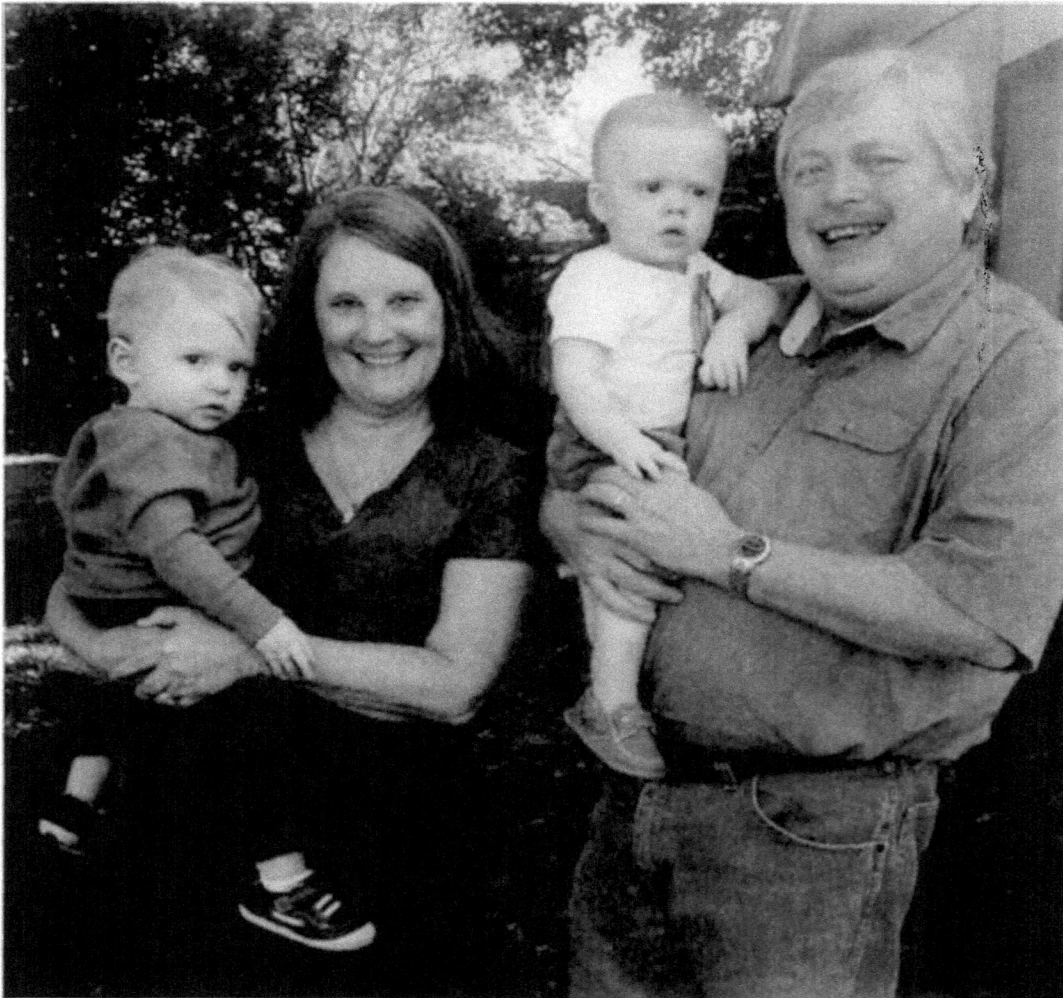

RANDALL EUGENE BRUCKMAN and PAMELA DENISE (BAILEY) BRUCKMAN

E3551 RAYMOND CLYDE LANTZ E355

RAYMOND CLYDE LANTZ was born on 20 Nov 1951 in Altoona, Blair Co., PA. He married (1) CHRISTINA IRENE LANTZ, 30 Aug 1969 in Duncansville, PA, daughter of ROBERT ALLEN LANTZ and ANNA DELL HUMERICK. She was born 16 Nov 1951 in Altoona, Blair Co., PA. They were divorced 09 Dec 1975, Hollidaysburg, Blair Co., PA; He married (2) DIANNA LEE CROSSLEY 26 Mar 1977 in Pensacola, Escambia Co., FL, daughter of NOEL NELSON CROSSLEY and SANDRA LEE SHAW. She was born 01 Nov 1956 in Pontiac, Oakland Co., MI. He served in the U.S. Navy 30 Apr 1969- 31 May 1989 and retired 29 Apr 1999. His current occupation is as a Software Engineer/Computer Programmer. DIANNA LEE CROSSLEY is a Native American with 1/4 Blood Degree of the Huron Potawatomi Tribe. He is the author of this book and currently resides at 8939 Abbington Drive, Pensacola, FL 32534-5347. He is a graduate of Embry Riddle Aeronautical University.

Child of RAYMOND LANTZ and CHRISTINA LANTZ is:

   i. YVONNE MARIE LANTZ (E35511)

Child of RAYMOND LANTZ and DIANNA CROSSLEY is:

   ii. NELSON GARFIELD LANTZ (E35512)

Ref: 24, 25, 27-B/RCL/199333-51/DOH PA, 27-B/DLC/6125/Oakland Co MI, 27-M/RCL&DLC/77-559/Escambia Co FL, 27-B/YML/1970/Prince George's Co MD, 27-M/RCL&CIL/73729/Blair Co PA, 27-DIV/RCL&CIL/530-1975/Blair Co PA, 19

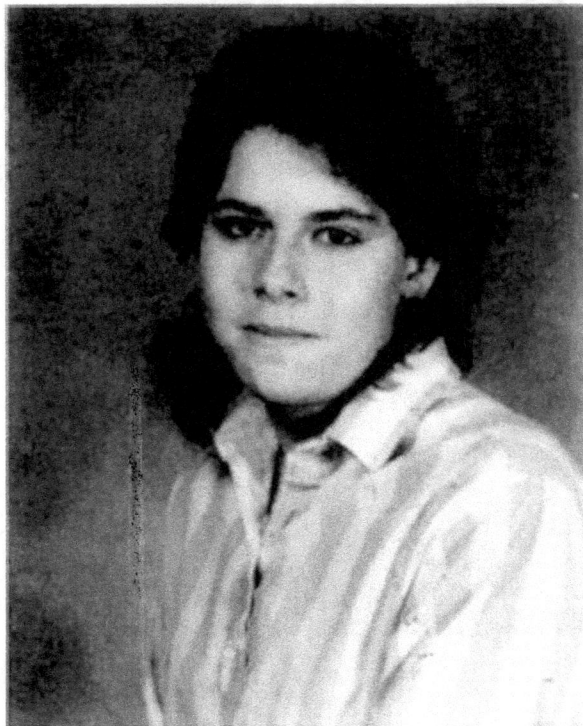

YVONNE MARIE LANTZ

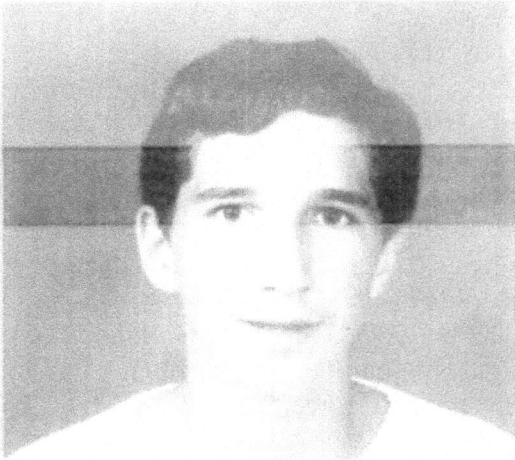

NELSON GARFIELD LANTZ

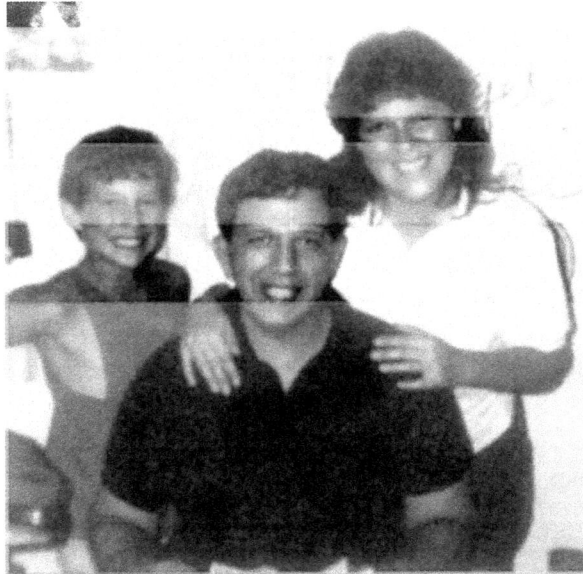

RAYMOND CLYDE, DIANNA LEE (CROSSLEY)
and NELSON GARFIELD LANTZ

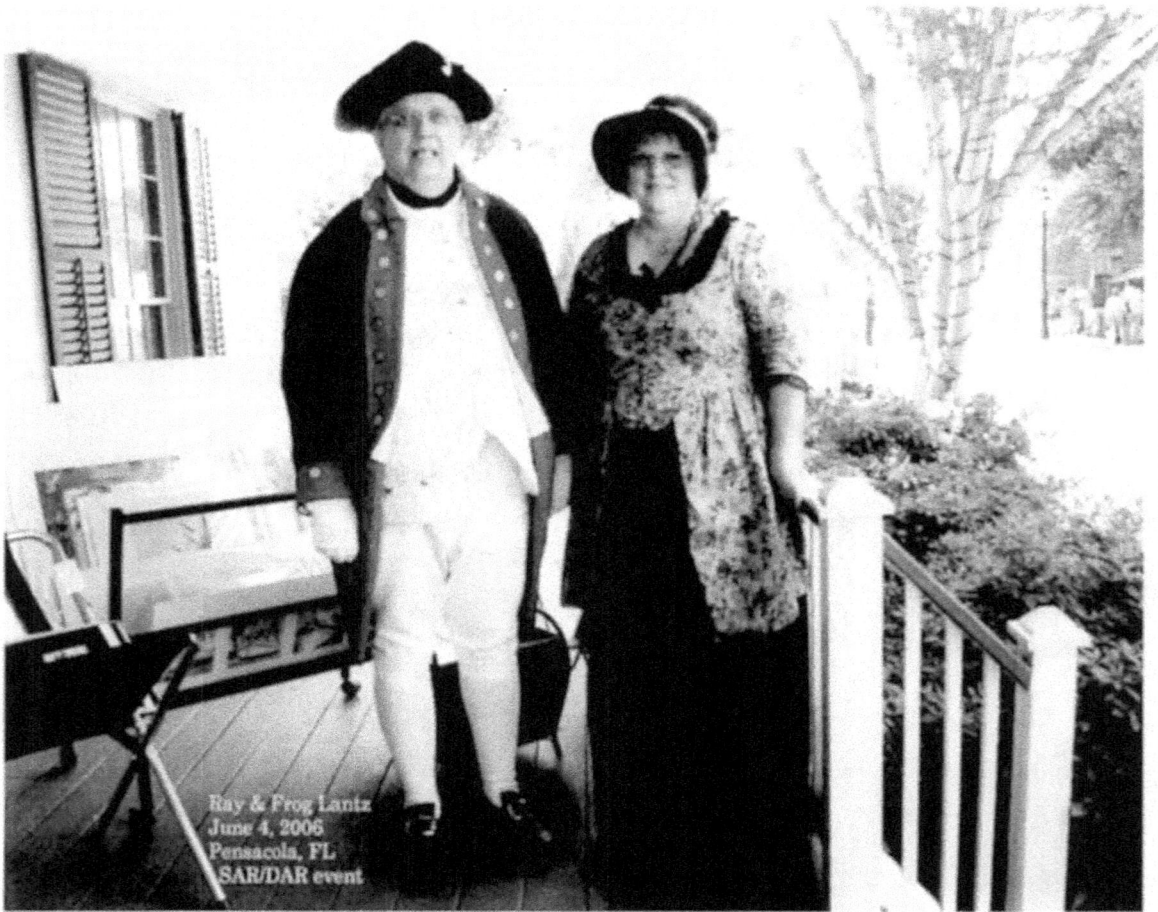

Ray & Frog Lantz
June 4, 2006
Pensacola, FL
SAR/DAR event

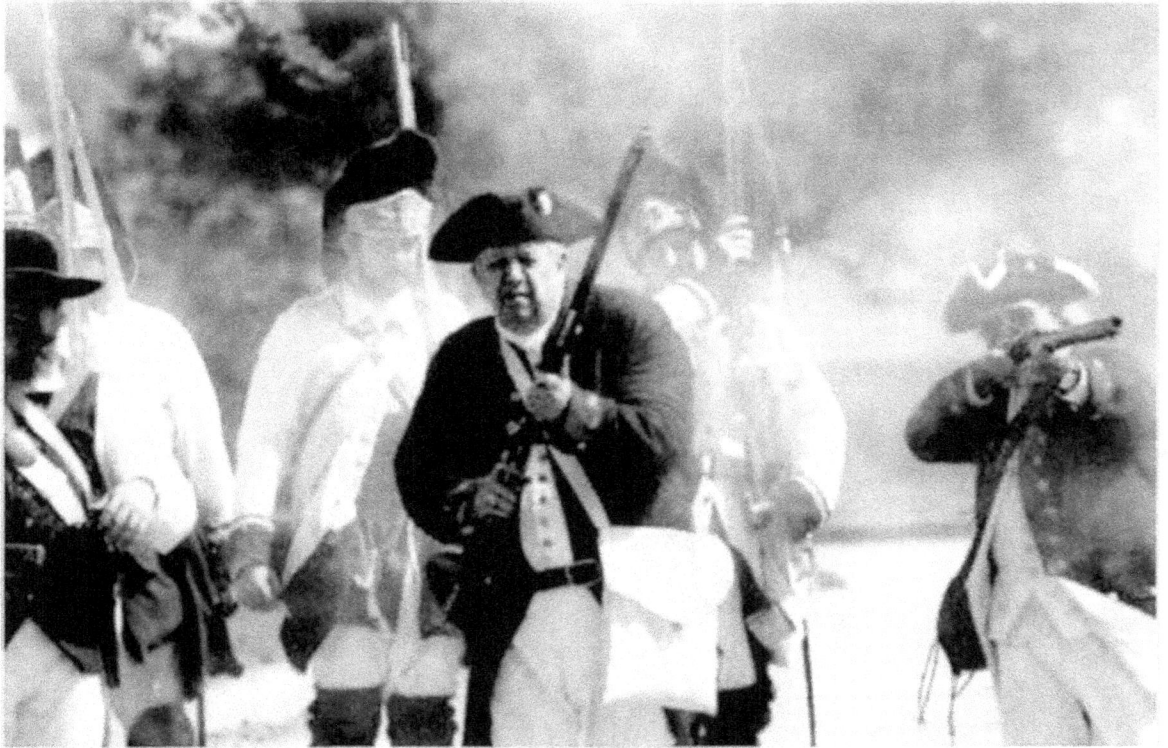

RAYMOND CLYDE LANTZ Battle of Pensacola Florida re-enactment

E3621 PEGGY GRIFFITH E362

PEGGY GRIFFITH was born on 19 Apr 1943 in WA. She married DANIEL J. COVERT on 20 Nov 1965 in WA, son of JOHN L. COVERT and LILLIAN GEDDES. He was born on 12 Mar 1941 in WA.

Children of PEGGY GRIFFITH and DANIEL COVERT are:

i. PAUL MICHAEL COVERT (E36211) was born in 11 Apr 1968 in IL.

ii. DAVID A. COVERT (E36212) was born on 09 Jun 1970 in WA.

Ref: 49, 23-William Richard Griffith

E3622 WILLIAM RICHARD GRIFFITH E362

WILLIAM RICHARD GRIFFITH was born on 19 Mar 1945 in WA. He married JULIE HASSELL on 04 Dec 1971 in _____, daughter of BROCK and EDNA (_____) HASSELL. She was born on 23 Feb 1950 in Renton, King Co., WA.

Children of WILLIAM GRIFFITH and JULIE HASSELL are:

i. JASON N. GRIFFITH (E36221)

ii. ZACHARY B. GRIFFITH (E36222)

iii. TIFFANY H. GRIFFITH (E36223) was born on 01 Aug 1978 in Edmonds, Snohomish Co., WA. She married LANCE RHOADES on 06 Jun 2003 in Seattle, King Co., WA, son of JEANNE (_____) RHOADES. He was born on 04 Mar 1968.

Ref: 49, 23-William Richard Griffith

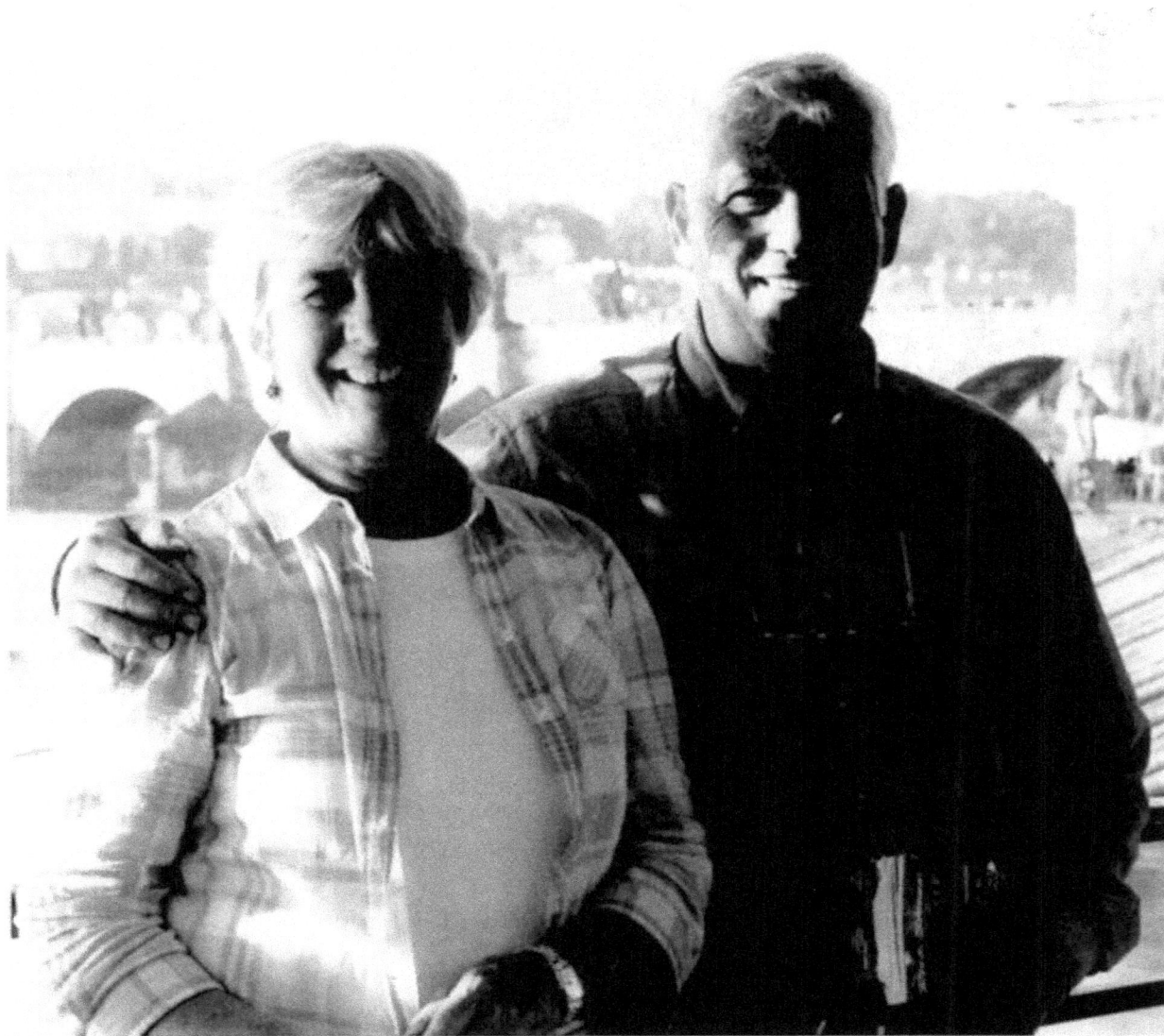

WILLIAM RICHARD and JULIE (HASSELL) GRIFFITH

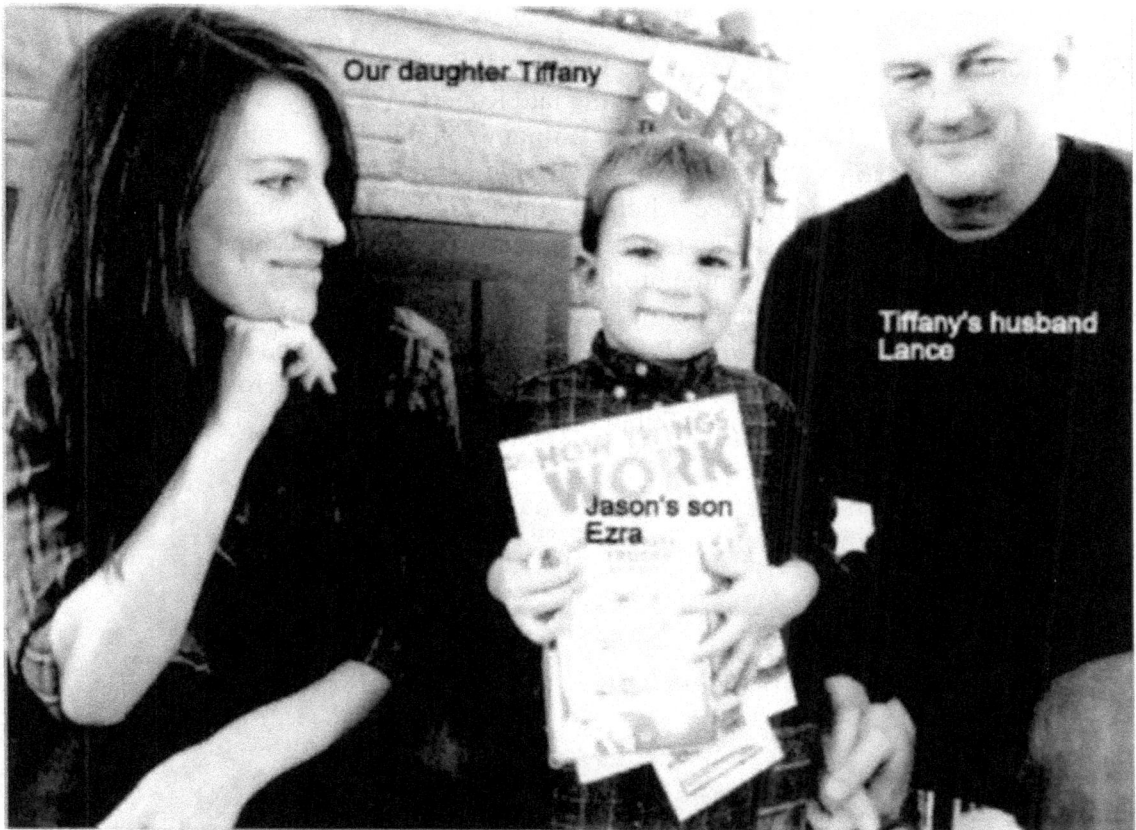

Our daughter Tiffany

Jason's son Ezra

Tiffany's husband Lance

E4123 GEORGE WILLIAM PETRY Jr. E412

GEORGE WILLIAM PETRY Jr. was born in 1927 in PA and died 06 Jan 2004 in Johnstown, Cambria Co., PA. He married LORRAINE M. JONES in PA, daughter of ROBERT MCKINLEY JONES and FLORENCE FARREL. She was born on 26 Dec 1928 in Wiota, Valley Co., MT. Both are buried in Forest Lawn Memorial Park, Johnstown, Cambria Co., PA.

Children of GEORGE PETRY and LORRAINE JONES are:

   i. ROBERT ALAN PETRY (E41231)

   ii. GEORGE WILLIAM PETRY III (E41232).

Ref: 26, 44, Brother's Obit

Name: PETRY, George W., Jr.
Died: 6 Jan 2004; Conemaugh Medical Center
Born: (age 76)
Spouse: Lorraine Jones (m. 54 yrs)
Prec. Death: Parents; brothers - Sanford & Eugene Petry
Survived By: Wife; children - Dr. Robert Petry (h/o Dr. Mary Loos); grandchildren - Skylar Petry, George W. Petry III (h/o Carol Allison), Melanie Petry, Dawn (w/o Keith Null); great-granddaughter - Allyson Rae Null; brothers – Melroy (h/o Eve), Robert (h/o Blanche); sisters-in-law - Hazel & Vivian Petry. Buried: Forest Lawn Cemetery
Newspaper: Tribune-Democrat 07 Jan 2004

PETRY – Lorraine M., 80, Johnstown, died Oct. 28, 2009, at Memorial Medical Center. Born Dec. 26, 1928, in Wiota, Mont., daughter of the late Robert McKinley and Florence (Farrel) Jones. Preceded in death by husband, George William Petry Jr.; five brothers; and a sister, all of Montana. Survived by sons, Dr. Robert Alan Petry, and wife, Dr. Mary (Loos), Richmond, Va.; George William Petry III, and fiancee, Michele Tomak, Johnstown; grandchildren, Melanie Petry, and fiance, Robert Owens; Dawn Null, and husband, Keith; and Skylar Petry; great-granddaughter, Allyson Rae Null; three brothers and three sisters, all of Montana; as well as numerous nieces and nephews. Member of Moxham Church of the Brethren. At the request of the deceased, there will be no viewing. Private memorial service will be held at Forest Lawn Cemetery, the Rev. William W. Wenger. John Henderson Co. Funeral Home.
Johnstown Tribune Democrat 31 Oct 2009

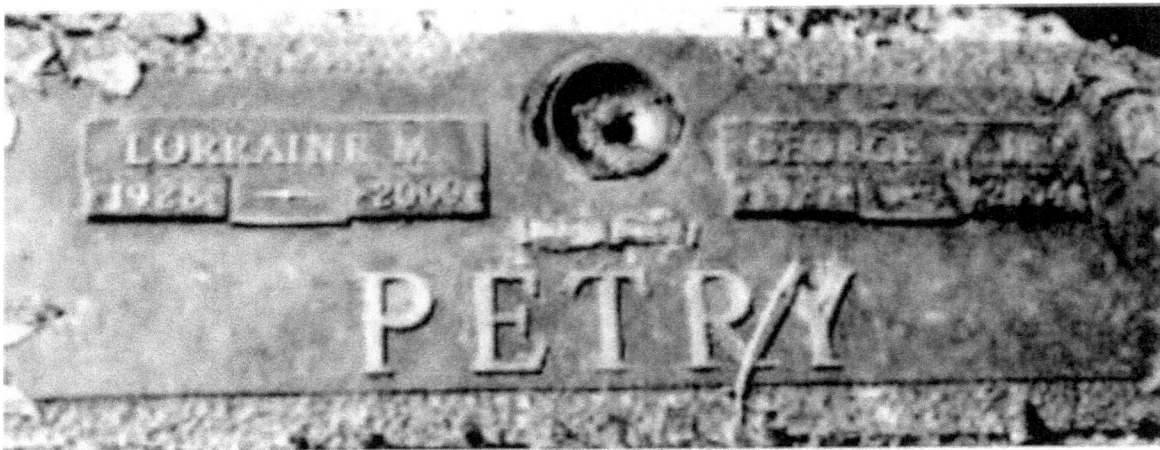

E4124 MELROY PETRY E412

MELROY "MELVIN" PETRY was born on 05 Sep 1929 in Johnstown, Cambria Co., PA and died 27 Dec 2014 in Port Saint Lucie, Saint Lucie Co., FL. He married EVA RLENE HOSTETLER, daughter of ELMER R. HOSTETLER and EDITH REBECCA DODGE.

i. JOEL PETRY (E41241) was born and died on 12 Apr 1960 in Johnstown, Cambria Co., PA.

ii. JOELENE PETRY (E41242) was born on 12 Apr 1960 and died 13 Apr 1960 in Johnstown, Cambria Co., PA.

iii. RENAE PETRY (E41242) was born in Johnstown, Cambria Co., PA.

Ref: 27-D-JP-35555, 27-D-JP-35556

MELROY (MEL) P. PETRY, 85, of Port Saint Lucie, FL, passed away December 27, 2014 in Port Saint Lucie, FL. Born September 5, 1929 in Johnstown, PA, son of George W. and Mazie (Shaffer) Petry. During the Korean War, Mel served in the Army. Prior to retirement, he was a bricklayer in the building industry. Mel is a member of Port Saint Lucie Christian Church and at one time had been a deacon. Survivors include his wife, Eva Petry and daughter, ReNae Petry of Port Saint Lucie, FL. Also his brother Robert Petry and wife Blanche along with two sisters-in-law, Hazel and Vivian Petry of Johnstown, PA. Preceded in death, brothers, Sanford, Eugene,

George and sister-in-law Lorraine Petry. Mel was loved deeply and will be greatly missed by wife and daughter. A Memorial Service will be held January 10, 2014 at Port Saint Lucie Christian Church, 1420 SE Floresta Drive, Port Saint Lucie, FL at 2PM.

http://www.aycockportstlucie.com

TC Palm 01 Jan. 2015

E4211 MARION V. DELOZIER E421

MARION V. DELOZIER was born in 1930 in Connellsville, Fayette Co., PA. She married LOYAL W. COWAN on 26 Jun 1949 in Connellsville, Fayette Co., PA, son of GEORGE A. COWAN. He was born on 11 May 1922 in Prospect, Cambria Co., PA and died 23 Jul 2009 in McAllen, Hidalgo Co., TX.

Children of MARION DELOZIER and LOYAL COWAN are:

i. CHRISTOPHER F. COWAN (E42111)

ii. SUSAN COWAN (E42112)

iii. CHARLOTTE COWAN (E42113)

iv. CURTIS COWAN (E42114)

Ref: 42

Loyal W. Cowan, 87, passed away on July 23, 2009, at Alfredo Gonzalez Veterans Home in McAllen, Texas. He was born in Prospect, Pa., on May 11, 1922. Loyal served in the U.S. Navy as a Machinist's Mate with the 91st Naval Construction Battalion (Seabees) in New Guinea and the Philippines from 1943-46. Surviving are his wife of 60 years, Marion, nee De Lozier; children, Christopher F. Cowan, Esq. (Anne Carrigg) of Dayton, Ohio, Susan (James W.) Johnston of Sapulpa, Okla., Charlotte (Erskine) Fulcher of Buxton, N.C., and Curtis (Monica) Cowan of East Hampton, Conn. Grandchildren are Claire Cowan, with the U.S. Navy, Mary Kroger and Christopher Loyal Cowan, Chicago, Eric Fulcher, Buxton, N.C., Eric Haury, Allison, and Lisa Clair Cowan, East Hampton, Conn., Jennie Tang, Jeff and Doug Johnston. Great-grandchildren are Emilie and Eric Fulcher, Jr., Buxton, N.C., and Josh Johnston, Dallas. Loyal's surviving siblings are brother, Raymond, Erie; and sisters, Bessie Smith, Mount Pleasant, and Bertha Brown, Ocala, Fla. His brother, Harold, preceded him in death. Loyal worked for Fruehauf Trailer Co. for 24 years and for the City of Elyria, Ohio, for 20 years. He was a charter member of Community United Methodist Church, Elyria, where he was an active worker for 35 years. Loyal loved being outdoors hiking, gardening and bird watching. In Ohio he was happy chopping wood for the fireplace and bragging about his big woodpile. At age 84 he was bicycling 10 to 15 miles every day. A memorial to Loyal will be held in Somerset in October. Donations can be sent to the Alzheimer's Association, 8546 Broadway St. San Antonio, TX 78217.

Daily American 27 July 2009

Marion DeLozier, Laboratory Technician, Wed at Church Ceremony to Loyal W. Cowan

Miss Marion V. DeLozier, daughter of Mr. and Mrs. Fred W. DeLozier, of Pittsburg street, South Connellsville, became the bride of Loyal W. Cowan, son of Mr. and Mrs. George A. Cowan, of Mount Pleasant, at a beautiful wedding Sunday afternoon in Trinity Evangelical and Reformed Church.

Rev. Paul Oberkircher, pastor of the church, performed the impressive double ring service at 3 o'clock in the presence of many relatives and friends. Marriage vows were repeated before an artistic arrangement of palms, ferns and a large basket of white gladioli.

Miss Leona Binkley of Englewood, Ohio, a former classmate of the bride at Ohio Institute, presided at the piano and presented a recital as the guests were assembling. Her program included "Because," "I Love You Truly," "Ah, Sweet Mystery of Life" and "Always." She played Wagner's "Bridal March" from "Lohengrin" as the wedding party came into the church.

Given in marriage by her father, the attractive bride wore a white sharkskin suit trimmed with pearl buttons, a pearl necklace, a gift from the bridegroom, a white horsehair sweetheart hat, white shoes and gloves. She carried a colonial bouquet of white roses and wore the traditional "something old, borrowed and blue." For good luck, she tucked a penny in the toe of her shoe.

The bride chose as her maid of honor and only attendant, a former High School friend, Miss Gloria Jean Smith, of South Connellsville. She wore a pink sharkskin suit, a white hat and corsage of cavalier roses.

Miss Binkley was attired in a pink dress and wore a corsage of yellow roses and blue delphinium.

Paul Wilson of Mount Pleasant, a friend of the bridegroom, was best man. Frank Simpson of Mount Pleasant, also a friend of the bridegroom, and William DeLozier of South Connellsville, brother of the bride, ushered.

After the wedding, a reception was held in the church. Seventy-five guests were present. The bride's table was adorned with a three-tiered wedding cake topped with a miniature bride and bridegroom.

The new Mrs. Cowan was graduated from Connellsville High School with the Class of 1947, attended Heidelberg College at Tiffin, Ohio, and graduated from Ohio Institute at Cleveland. She is a laboratory technician at Allen Hospital, Oberlin, Ohio.

The bridegroom is employed by Fruehoff Trailer Company at Avon Lake, Ohio.

The newlyweds left for a wedding trip to Niagara Falls and Canada. They will be at home July 5 at 221 North Professor street, Oberlin, Ohio.

Out-of-town guests at the wedding were from Ravenna, Ohio, McDonald, Houston, Tex., Pittsburgh, Somerset, Mount Pleasant, Butler, Washington, Glencoe and Monongahela.

The Daily Courier 30 Jun 1949

128

E4221 MARIETTA L. SMITH E422

MARIETTA L. SMITH was born on 06 Dec 1921 in Meyersdale, Somerset Co., PA and died 26 Jun 2003 in Somerset, Somerset Co., PA. She married MILTON E. GIFFIN in Somerset Co., PA. He was born on 17 Apr 1918 in Boswell, Somerset Co., PA and died 31 Jul 1999 in Somerset, Somerset Co., PA.

Children of MARIETTA SMITH and MILTON GIFFIN are:

  i. DARLENE L. GIFFIN (E42211)

  ii. MILTON BARRY GIFFIN (E42212)

Ref: 44

Marietta L. (Smith) Giffin, 81 of Boswell, died June 26, 2003 at Somerset Hospital. Born Dec. 6, 1921 in Meyersdale a daughter of Dewey and Alma (deLozier) Smith. Preceded in death by parents; husband of 56 years, Milton E. on July 31, 1999, son-in-law Larry Benshoff, and brother Chester Smith. Survived by daughter, Darlene L. Benshoff of Erie; son, Milton Barry married to former Diana "Dee" Unger of Collegeville; grandsons, Brian and Jeffrey Benshoff and Eric Giffin; stepgranddaughters, Tina Dean, and Tami Barnes; stepgreat-grandsons, Gunnar and Troy Dean; sisters, Helen widow of Ray Weigle of Friedens, Roberta Ling-Kaulp Mansfield Ohio and Emma Jean married to Ray Charlton of Hollidaysburg and sister-in-law Rose (Kozel) Smith of Acosta. Also survived by numerous nieces and nephews. Member of the Boswell Church of God. She enjoyed knitting, reading and singing with her family. Friends received from 2 to 4 and 7 to 9 p.m. Saturday at Hoffman Funeral Home Allegheny St., Boswell ,where a service will be held 1 p.m. Sunday. The Rev. Gregory Stauffer officiating. Interment, Jenner Crossroads Cemetery. Memorial donations in Marietta's name may be sent to the Boswell Church of God, Main Street, Boswell, Pa. 15531.

Daily American 27 Jun 2003

Milton E. Giffin, 81, of Allegheny Street, Boswell, died July 31, 1999, at Somerset Hospital. Born April 17, 1918, in Boswell. Preceded in death by father, Earl S. Giffin, and mother Ethel Mae (Rice) Giffin-Mickol, stepfather, John Mickol, and sister, Alice Shaffer. Survived by wife, the former Marietta L. Smith; children, Darlene L. Benshoff, Erie, Milton Barry, married to former Diana "Dee" Unger, Collegeville; grandsons, Brian and Jeffrey Benshoff and Eric Scott Giffin; also numerous nieces and nephews. Attended Boswell Church of God. Former member of Jenner Rod & Gun Club. Observed 56th wedding anniversary Jan. 17, 1999. Retired Crane Director for Bethlehem Steel Corporation, Johnstown Works with over 37 years service. Avid hunter and fisherman. Also enjoyed playing various musical instruments and was a member of several local bands through the years. Friends received from 2-4 and 7-9 p.m., Monday at Hoffman Funeral Home, Allegheny Street, Boswell, where service will be held at 11 a.m., Tuesday, Rev. Gregory Stauffer officiating. Interment Jenner Cross Roads Cemetery. Memorial contributions may be sent to Boswell Church of God, Main Street, Boswell, Pa. 15531.

Daily American 02 Aug 1999

E4223 HELEN E. SMITH E422

HELEN E. SMITH was born in Somerset Co., PA. She married RAY T. WEIGLE in Somerset Co., PA, son of HARVEY M. WEIGLE and CLARA SUDER. He was born on 17 Oct 1924 in Stonycreek Twp., Somerset Co., PA and died 20 Sep 1997 in Somerset, Somerset Co., PA.

Child of HELEN SMITH and RAY WEIGLE is:

   i. R. LYNN WEIGLE (E42231)

Ref: 44

Ray T. Weigle, 72, of Sand Rock Road, Friedens, died Sept. 20, 1997 at Patriot Manor, Somerset. Born Oct. 17, 1924, in Stonycreek Township, son of Harvey M. and Clara (Suder) Weigle. Preceded in death by parents; brothers: Glenn, Melvin, William, Ernest and Nevin; sisters: Ethel Onstead and Myrtie Fritz. Survived by his wife of 52 years, the former Helen Smith; son, R. Lynn, married to former Esther Mostoller, Friedens; grandson, Jeremy Lynn. Brother of Harry, Berlin, and Pauline Baumgardner, Friedens. A retired salesman for Servos Seed Co. and Furst-McNess Co. A World War II Army veteran. Member of Faith Lutheran Church. Member and former master of Somerset Grange. Also member of county, state and national Granges; Shanksville American Legion Post 911 and DAV. Family received friends Sunday evening and will receive friends from 2 to 4 and 7 to 9 p.m. Monday at Deaner Funeral Home, Stoystown. Viewing from 10 a.m. until service at 11 a.m. Tuesday at Faith Lutheran Church, Rev. Randall Marburger officiating. Interment, Somerset County Memorial Park. Memorial contributions may be given to Faith Lutheran Church, Glades Pike, Somerset, Pa, 15501. Graveside military rites by Menoher Post 155 VFW Ritual Team.

Daily American 22 Sep 1997

E4225 EMMA JEAN SMITH E422

EMMA JEAN SMITH was born on 03 Feb 1938 in Boswell, Somerset Co., PA and died 15 Aug 2004 in Altoona, Blair Co., PA. She married JASON RAY CHARLTON in Somerset Co., PA, son of SAMUEL CHARLTON and VERGIE DOVE. He was born on 11 Oct 1940 in Somerset Co., PA and died 09 Aug 2013 in Hollidaysburg, Blair Co., PA.

Child of EMMA SMITH and JASON CHARLTON is:

   i. DAVID J. CHARLTON (E4225) married AMY RENEE BERKHEIMER.

Ref: 44

Emma Jean Charlton

Mrs. Emma Jean Charlton, 66, of Hollidaysburg, formerly of Boswell and Somerset, died Aug. 15, 2004, at Bon Secours-Holy Family Hospital. She was born Feb. 3, 1938, in Boswell, the daughter of the late Dewey and Alma (Delozier) Smith. She married Jason "Ray" Charlton Dec. 24, 1966.

She is survived by her husband; a son, David J. and fiancee, Amy Renee Berkheimer, of Hollidaysburg; and sisters: Helen, widow of Ray Weigle, of Friedens, and Roberta Ling-Kaulp of Mansfield, Ohio; numerous nieces and nephews; and other relatives. Mrs. Charlton was preceded in death by her parents; a sister, Marietta Giffin; and a brother, Chester A. She was a 1955 graduate of the former JBJ Joint High School, Boswell. Mrs. Charlton was a former employee of Selected Risks, Somerset. She was a member of Hollidaysburg Church of God. Friends will be received from 7 to 9 p.m. Tuesday and noon to the 2 p.m. service Wednesday at Hoffman Funeral Home, Main Street, Boswell (814-629-5550). Interment will be at Odd Fellows Cemetery, Stoystown.

Altoona Mirror 16 Aug 2004

Jason Ray Charlton, 72, Hollidaysburg, formerly of Somerset County, died Aug. 9, 2013, at the home of son David. Born Oct. 11, 1940, in Somerset County, son of Samuel and Vergie (Dove) Charlton. Preceded in death by parents; wife of 38 years, former Emma Jean Smith on Aug. 15, 2004; and brothers: the Rev. Samuel, Vincent, Franklin and Fred. Survived by son David, married to Amy Renee Berkheimer, Hollidaysburg; sister Dorothy Corden; and sister-in-law Betty Charlton. Also numerous nieces and nephews. Graduate of former Forbes High School and retired retail manager for Woolworth's stores. Viewing 11 a.m. until time of service 1 p.m. Monday at Hoffman Funeral Home & Cremation Services, 409 Main St., Boswell, Pastor Larry C. Hoover officiating. Interment Odd Fellows Cemetery, Stoystown. For further information visit hoffmanfuneralhomes.com

Daily American 11 Aug 2013

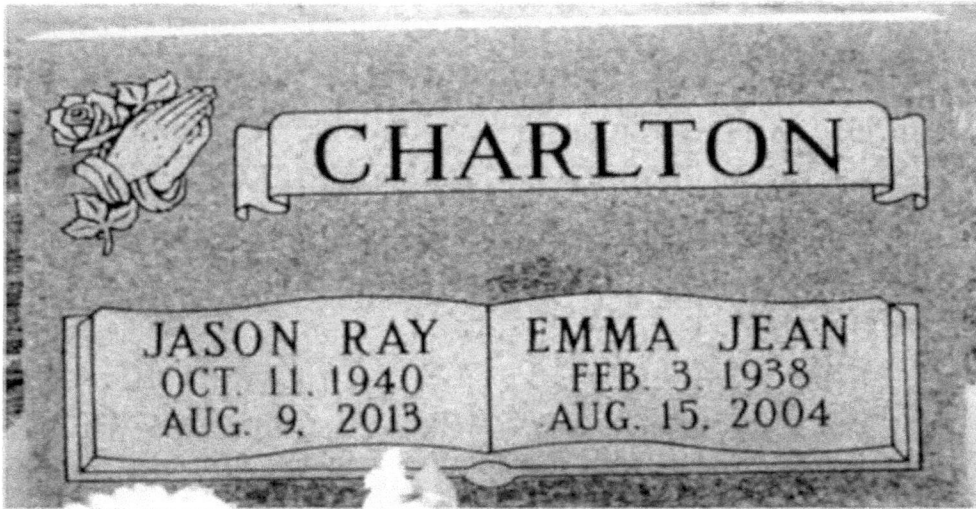

E4254 MAXINE J. DELOZIER E425

MAXINE J. DELOZIER was born in Somerset Co., PA. She married ALBERT D. FUREDY Sr.

Children of MAXINE DELOZIER and ALBERT FUREDY are:

i. ALBERT D. FUREDY Jr. (E42541) was born in 1966 in PA and died 23 Jul 2014 in Pittsburgh, Allegheny Co., PA.

FUREDY ALBERT D., Jr.
Age 48, of Mount Lebanon, unexpectedly on Wednesday, July 23, 2014. Dearly beloved son of Albert D., Sr. and Maxine J. (DeLozier) Furedy; loving brother of Karen E. (Michael) Veith, Steven P. (Becki) Furedy and David R. (Marie) Furedy; cherished uncle of Ryan, Kayla and Brooke Veith, Ella, Kenny and Andrew Furedy; beloved nephew of Frances A. Furedy, Janet (Jim) Stoops of Cumberland, MD, Barbara A. Furedy and Ruth Furedy; dear friend of Donna Wagner; also survived by his furry companion, Boo; many cousins and friends. Al loved gardening, cooking, fishing and was a loving friend to all who knew him. Visitation Saturday 12-5 p.m. with private family service at 6 p.m. at WILLIAM SLATER II FUNERAL SERVICE, (412-563-2800) 1650 Greentree Rd., Scott Twp. In lieu of flowers, memorials may be made to Animal Friends, 562 Camp Horne Rd., Pgh., PA 15237. www.slaterfuneral.com Send condolences post-gazette.com/gb
Pittsburgh Post-Gazette 25-26 July 2014

ii. KAREN E. FUREDY (E42542)

iii. STEVEN P. FUREDY (E42543) was born 29 Mar 1970 in PA. He married BECKI _____.

iv. DAVID R. FUREDY (E42544) was born 22 Nov 1975 in PA. He married MARIE _____.

Ref: 44, 49

E4262 DALE F. LUDY E426

DALE F. LUDY was born in 22 Aug 1934 in Glencoe, Somerset Co., PA and died 02 Nov 1999 in Seminole, Seminole Co., FL. He married JANICE ROBBINS. He is buried in Mt. Lebanon Cemetery, Glencoe, Somerset Co., PA.

Children of DALE LUDY and JANICE ROBBINS are:

   i. STACY LUDY (E42621)

   ii. DALE LUDY (E42622)

   iii. JEFFREY LUDY (E42623)

Ref: 44

Dale F. Ludy, 65, of Seminole, Fla., formerly of Berlin, died Nov. 2, 1999, in Seminole. Born Aug. 22, 1934, in Glencoe. Son of the late James Erwin and Emma Edith (DeLozier) Ludy. Survived by his wife, the former Janice Robbins, and these children: Stacy Bruning of Anchorage, Alaska; Dale of Seminole, and Jeffrey of New Port Richey, Fla.; grandchildren, Arin and Sara Bruning, Nicholas and Alexis Ludy. Brother of Wayne Miller of Greenwood, Ind., James Ludy of Mechanicsburg, and Mary Kreinbrook of Berlin. Retired from the U.S. Air Force. Memorial service will be held at 3 p.m. Saturday at Deaner Funeral Home, Berlin. Rev. Melvin A. Kirk, Jr. Interment; Mt. Lebanon Cemetery, Glencoe.
Daily American 04 Nov 1999

E4321 JACK A. HENRY E432

JACK A. HENRY was born on 1924 in Somerset Co., PA and died 26 Mar 1985 in Keyser, Mineral Co., WV. He married GENEVIEVE GRACE THOMAS in Somerset Co., PA. He is buried in Rest Lawn Memorial Gardens, LaVale, Allegany Co., MD.

Children of JACK HENRY and GENEVIEVE THOMAS are:

   i. GEORGE ALLEN HENRY (E43211)

   ii. JAMES ROBERT HENRY (E43212)

   iii. THOMAS CHARLES HENRY (E43213)

Ref: 44, 49

Jack Allen Henry, 61, of 185 West Piedmont Street, Keyser, West Virginia, died Tuesday, March 26, 1985, at his residence. He was born in Meyersdale, a son of Mrs. Anna J. (Sharp) Henry, Meyersdale, and the late Charles F. Henry. He was retired in 1978 as a track inspector for the Chessie System. He was a member of Grace United Methodist Church; David Lodge 51, AF&AM, and the Senior Citizens of Mineral County. Besides his mother, he is survived by his widow, the former Genevieve Thomas; three sons, George A. Henry, Barton; James R. Henry, at home; Thomas C. Henry, Keyser; one brother, Harold H. Henry, Aliquippa, and four grandchildren. Friends were received at the Markwood-McKenzie Funeral Home chapel where services were conducted by the Rev. David R. Peters. Interment Rest Lawn Memorial Gardens, LaVale, Md.

The Republic 04 Apr 1985

E4821 LESLIE H. MULL E482

LESLIE H. MULL was born in 1939 in Somerset Co., PA. He married MICHELLE L. _____.

Children of LESLIE MULL and MICHELLE _____ are:

i. LESLIE H. MULL II (E48211)

ii. ERIC A. MULL (E48212)

iii. RHONDA MICHELLE MULL (E48213)

Ref: 44

E4231 JAMES E. HARTMAN E423

JAMES E. HARTMAN was born in 05 Mar 1924 in Glencoe, Somerset Co., PA and died 15 Jul 1996 in Pittsburgh, Allegheny Co., PA. He married VIRGINIA M. GRENKE, daughter of JOHN F. GRENKE and MARIA PEARL EGOLF. He was buried Mount Lebanon Cemetery, Glencoe, Somerset Co., PA.

Children of JAMES HARTMAN and are:

i. DAVID B. HARTMAN (E42311) married MARY ANN _____.

ii. DENNIS W. HARTMAN (E42312) married KATHY _____.

iii. DONNA L. HARTMAN (E42313)

Ref: 44

U.S. World War II Army Enlistment Records, 1938-1946
Name: James E Hartman
Birth Year: 1924
Race: White, citizen (White)
Nativity State or Country: Pennsylvania
State of Residence: Pennsylvania
County or City: Somerset
Enlistment Date: 29 Jan 1943
Enlistment State: Pennsylvania
Enlistment City: Altoona

Branch Code: Branch Immaterial - Warrant Officers, USA
Grade: Private
Grade Code: Private
Term of Enlistment: Enlistment for the duration of the War or other emergency, plus six
months, subject to the discretion of the President or otherwise according to law
Component: Selectees (Enlisted Men)
Source: Civil Life
Education: 4 years of high school
Civil Occupation: Semiskilled occupations in building of aircraft, n.e.c.
Marital Status: Single, without dependents
Height: 72
Weight: 170

James E. Hartman, 72, of Lincoln Street, Somerset, died July 15, 1996, at Allegheny General
Hospital, Pittsburgh. Born March 5, 1924, in Glencoe. Son of the late John W. and Mary M.
(DeLozier) Hartman. Survived by his wife of 50 years, the former Virginia M. Grenke; and two
sons, David B. Hartman, Canfield, Ohio; and Dennis W. Hartman, Washington, Pa.; and one
daughter, Donna L. Hartman, Brigantine, N.J. Also, grandson Wesley Scott Hartman and
granddaughters Jamie Marie and Kristy Hartman. Retired Penelec line foreman. Member of St.
Paul's United Church of Christ. Past master of Somerset Lodge No. 358 F&AM, where he
served as member, trustee and president of the Temple Board and Ritual Instructor. Member of
Harrisburg Consistory and Jaffa Shrine of Altoona. WWII Veteran of Army Air Corps and
member of Somerset American Legion, where he served as past commander and temple board
member. Very active with the youth of the area and instrumental in forming the Little and the
Senior Baseball leagues, where he served as manager and a coach. He was cub master of Troop
131 of Somerset. Member of the Last Man's Club of Berlin. Honorary member of the Somerset
Fire Department. Avid golfer. Friends will be received from 7-9 p.m. Wednesday (today) and 2-
4 and 7-9 p.m. Thursday at the Wilbur D. Miller Funeral Home, Somerset. Funeral service will
be conducted at St. Paul's United Church of Christ at 11 a.m. Friday, with Rev. Glenn Sadler
officiating. Masonic services 7:30 p.m., Thursday at the funeral home. Interment at Mount
Lebanon Cemetery, Glencoe. There will be no viewing of the remains at the church.

Daily American 17 Jul 1996

Virginia M. Hartman, 80, Austintown, Ohio, formerly of Somerset, passed on May 25, 2004, at
Alterra - Clarebridge Cottage Personal Care Home. Born May 4, 1924, in Brothersvalley
Township, she is the daughter of the late John F. and Maria Pearl (Egolf) Grenke. She is
preceded in death by her parents; husband, James E. Hartman in 1996 and brothers, Frederick
and John Grenke. Also survived by brother Telford Grenke, Conway, S.C. She is survived by
her children, David, married to Mary Ann, Hartman, Canfield, Ohio; Dennis, married to Kathy,
Hartman, Washington and Donna Hartman Pless, married to Robert, Egg Harbor, N.J.; and
grandchildren, Wesley, Jamie and Kristy Hartman. She was a member of St. Paul's United
Church of Christ, Somerset. Friends may call from 5 to 9 p.m. Thursday at Miller Funeral Home,
Somerset where service will be held 11 a.m. Friday. The Rev. Dr. Herbert Hicks officiating.
Interment Mt. Lebanon Cemetery in Glencoe.

Daily American 27 May 2004

E4274 CONNIE DELOZIER E427

CONNIE DELOZIER was born on 12 Apr 1941 and died 12 Mar 2007 in Hancock, Washington Co., MD. She married THOMAS LEROY WINEBRENNER. He was born on 09 Jan 1940. She is buried in Frostburg Memorial Park, Frostburg, Allegany Co., MD.

Child of CONNIE DELOZIER and THOMAS WINEBRENNER is:

    i. THOMAS LEROY WINEBRENNER II (E42741)

Ref: 49, 42, 26

HANCOCK - Connie D. Winebrenner, 65, of Hancock, died Monday, March 12, 2007, at Johns Hopkins Hospital in Baltimore. She was born April 12, 1941, in Wellersburg, Pa. She was a member of Hancock United Methodist Church, where she sang in the choir and was active in various church activities. She was a graduate of Mount Savage High School, Mount Savage, Md., and retired after 35 years of service as Branch Manager with Susquehanna Bank in Hancock. She was a member of Berkeley Chapter 77 Order of the Eastern Star. She enjoyed bowling and had been a homemaker in recent years. She is survived by her husband of 44 years, Thomas LeRoy Winebrenner, at home; one son, Thomas LeRoy Winebrenner II, Frederick; two grandsons, Sean Thomas Winebrenner and Dylan Patrick Winebrenner, both of Frederick. She was preceded in death by her parents. Memorial services will be conducted Monday, March 19, 2007, at 10 a.m. in Hancock United Methodist Church, 170 W. Main St., Hancock, with the Rev. Duane Jensen officiating. Private interment will be in Frostburg Memorial Park, Frostburg. Arrangements are being handled by the Helsley-Johnson Funeral Home, 95 Union St., Berkeley Springs, WV.

Morning Herald, The/The Daily Mail 16 Mar 2007

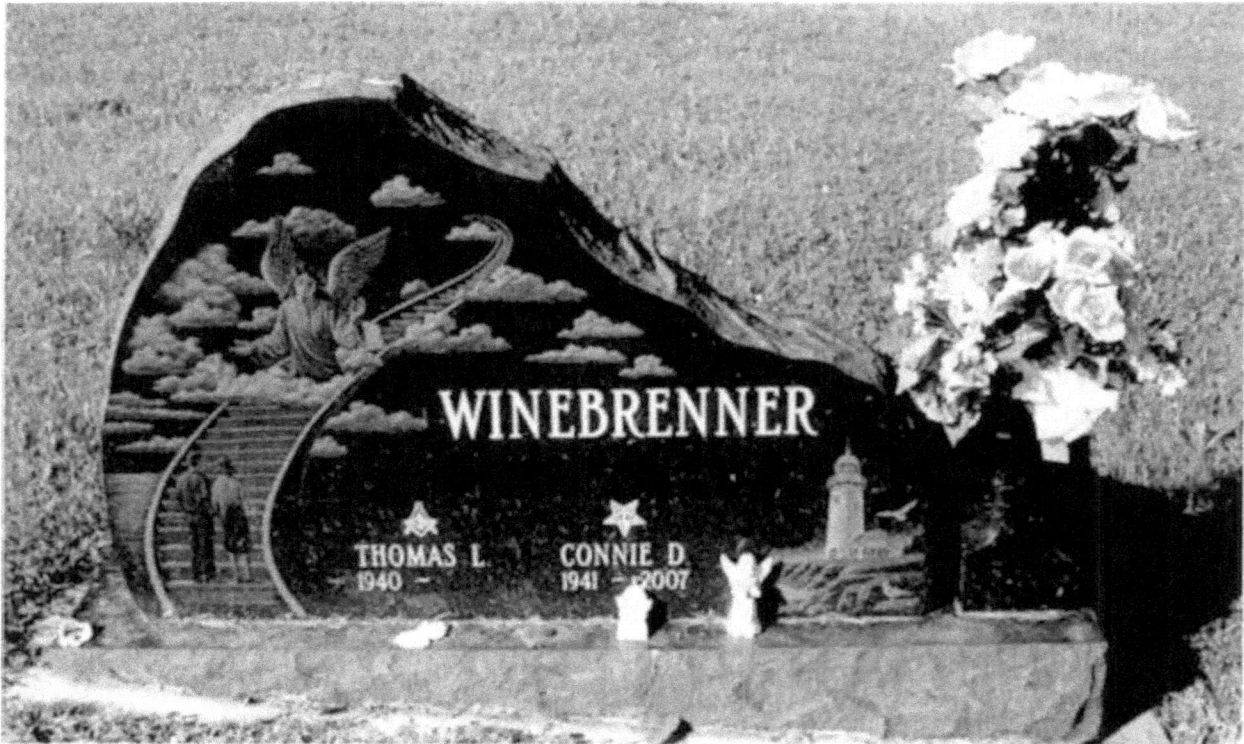

E4275 SHEILA R. DELOZIER E427

SHEILA R. DELOZIER was born on 24 Dec 1949. She married BRADLEY JOSEPH DENSOCK.

Child of SHEILA DELOZIER and BRADLEY DENSOCK is:

  i. BRETT JOSEPH DENSOCK (E42751) married MICHELE _____.

Ref: 44, 49

E4331 CLYDE IRVIN HOUSEL E433

CLYDE IRVIN HOUSEL was born on 05 Aug 1923. He married ADALINE CHRISTINI BURNETT, daughter of _____ BURNETT and _____ MCMILLAN. She was born on 22 Mar 1931 in Youngstown, Mahoning Co., OH and died 07 Nov 1997 in Elyria, Lorain Co., OH. She is buried in Sarasota National Cemetery, Sarasota, Sarasota Co., FL.

Child of CLYDE HOUSEL and ADALINE CHRISTINI is:

  i. ROBERT ALLEN HOUSEL (E43311)

Ref: 44, 49, 26, 59, 48, 42

U.S. World War II Army Enlistment Records, 1938-1946
Name: Clyde I Housel
Birth Year: 1923
Race: White, citizen (White)
Nativity State or Country: Pennsylvania
State of Residence: Ohio
County or City: Mahoning
Enlistment Date: 15 Mar 1943
Enlistment State: Ohio
Enlistment City: Fort Hayes Columbus
Branch: No branch assignment
Branch Code: No branch assignment
Grade: Private
Grade Code: Private
Term of Enlistment: Enlistment for the duration of the War or other emergency, plus six months, subject to the discretion of the President or otherwise according to law
Component: Selectees (Enlisted Men)
Source: Civil Life
Education: 4 years of high school
Civil Occupation: Semiskilled chauffeurs and drivers, bus, taxi, truck, and tractor
Marital Status: Single, without dependents
Height: 44
Weight: 122

E4843 SIDNEY GEORGE MULL E484

SIDNEY GEORGE MULL was born Monroeville, PA and died 19 Jul 2007 in Johnstown, Cambria Co., PA. He married ELLEN HOUSEL in PA.

Children of SIDNEY MULL and ELLEN HOUSEL are:

    i. JOHN CHARLES MULL (E48431)

    ii. SIDNEY GEORGE MULL Jr. (E48432)

    iii. CHANTAY ELIZABETH MULL (E48433)

    iv. TONYA YVONNE MULL (E48434)

Ref: 44

Sidney George "Bud" Mull Sr., 63, Salisbury, died July 19, 2007, at Memorial Medical Center, Johnstown. Born Feb. 2, 1944, in Monroeville, a son of the late Sidney Fay and Florence Maxine (Menhorn) Mull. He is preceded in death by one brother, Allen Wayne Mull. Surviving are his wife, Ellen (Housel) Mull; two sons, John Charles Mull and friend, Paula, Wellersburg; Sidney G. "B.J." Mull Jr. and friend, Melody, Salisbury; two daughters, Chantay Elizabeth Lawson and husband, Michael, Friendsville, Md.; Tonya Yvonne Christner and husband, Kenneth, Meyersdale; one stepson, Jeff Gray and wife, Lori, Salisbury; one stepdaughter, Beth Anne Brown and friend, Sean, Meyersdale; one brother, Donald Raymond Mull and wife, Mary Lee, Mayer, Ariz.; two sisters, Joyce Eileen McGhee, Holt, Mich.; Brenda Kay Haning and husband Freeman, St. Paul; and 12 grandchildren, Cody Twigg, Charlene Mull, Catharine Lawson, Robert Lawson, Kenneth Christner III, Tiffani Christner, Tori Christner, Triniti Christner, Tiani Christner, Brooke Gray, Liliana Shumaker and Ella Rose Mull. Mr. Mull was employed as a bricklayer with Local 15 BAC. He is a U.S. Army veteran of the Vietnam War and a member of Salisbury American Legion Post 459. He was a member of the Maple Leaf Rod and Gun Club, Kennells Mill Outdoor Club, Barrelville Outdoor Club and St. John's United Church of Christ. Friends will be received 7 to 9 p.m. Saturday and 2 to 4 and 7 to 9 p.m. Sunday at the Newman Funeral Home Inc., 9168 Mason-Dixon Highway, Salisbury, where a service will be conducted 2 p.m. Monday. The Rev. David E. Fetter officiating. Interment will be in Salisbury Cemetery, where military graveside rites will be accorded by Salisbury American Legion Post 459. Expressions of sympathy may be directed to Salisbury American Legion Post 459, Scholarship Fund. Condolences may be sent to the family at www.newman-funeralhomes. com.

Daily American 20 Jul 2007

E35311 TERRY RAYMOND BRUCKMAN E3531

TERRY RAYMOND BRUCKMAN was born on 30 Apr 1972. He married KIMBERLY "KIM" DAWN COLE on 07 Aug 1993 in Memphis, Shelby Co., TN.

Children of TERRY BRUCKMAN and KIMBERLY COLE are:

i. BRADLEY "BRAD" THOMAS BRUCKMAN (E353111) was born on 22 Nov 2000 in Memphis, Shelby Co., TN.

ii. BRANDON COLE BRUCKMAN(E353112) was born on 12 Jun 2002 in Memphis, Shelby Co., TN.

Ref: 23-Wendi Lynn Bruckman

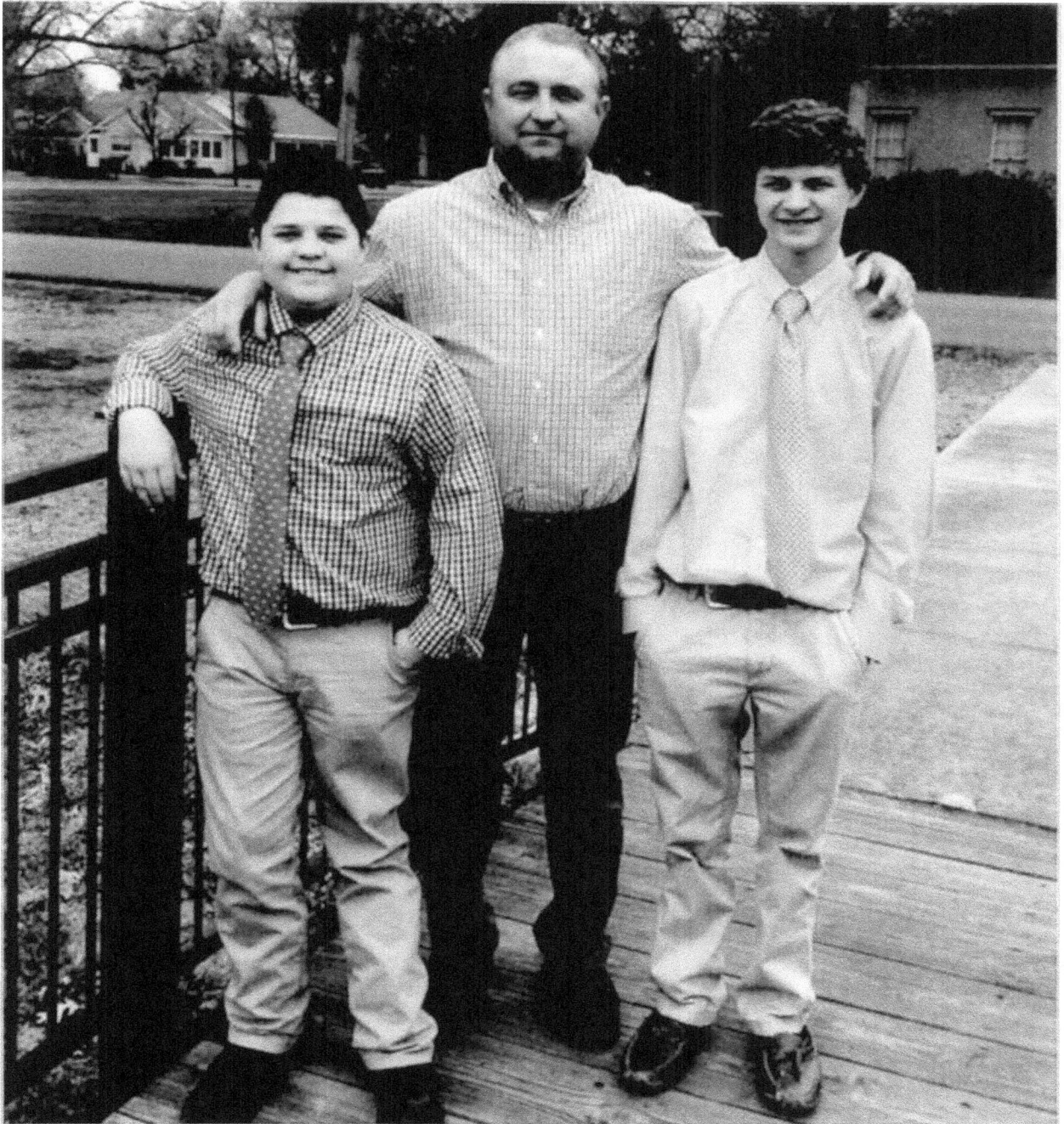

BRANDON COLE, TERRY RAYMOND and BRADLEY THOMAS BRUCKMAN

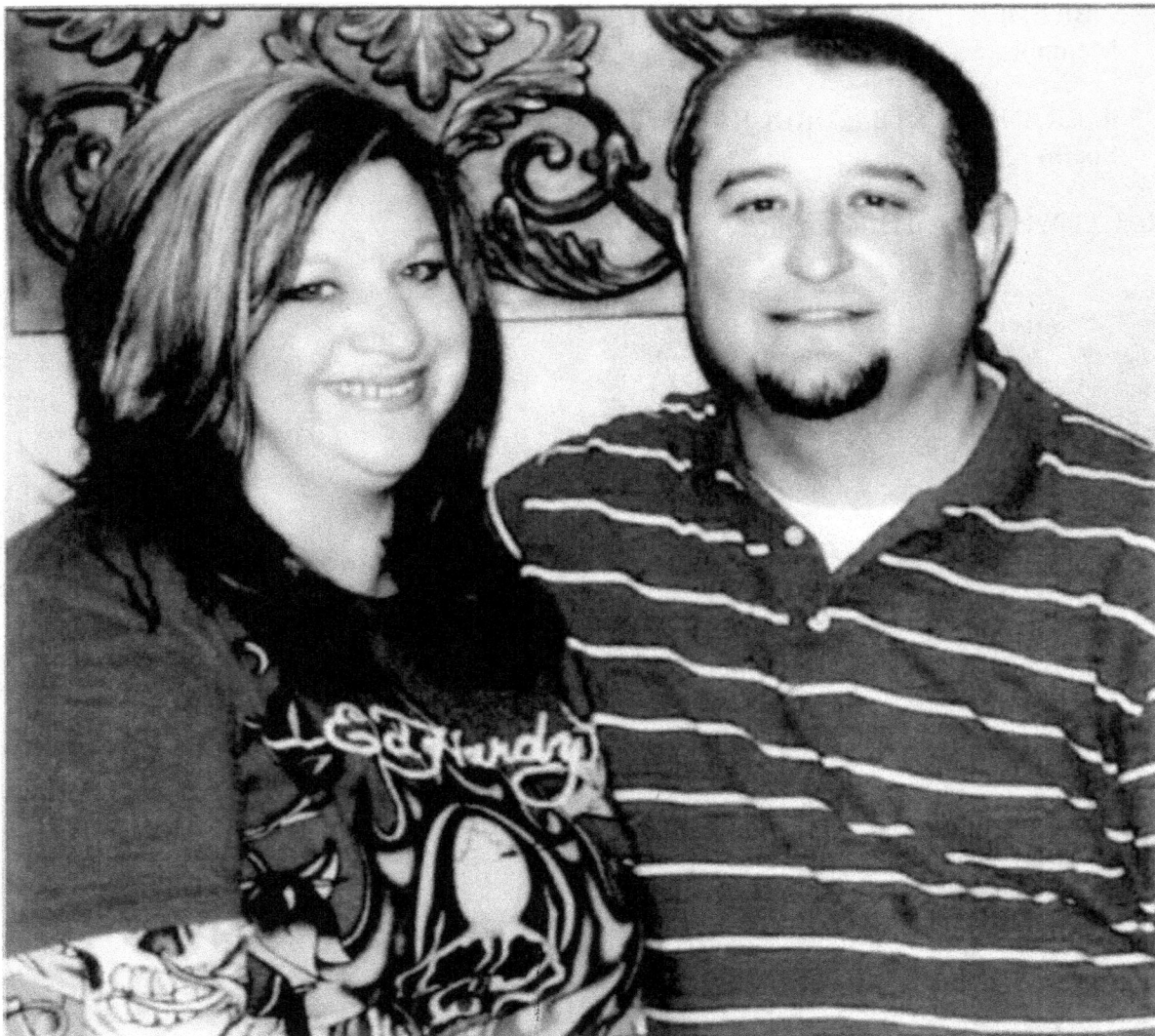

TERRY RAYMOND and KIMBERLY DAWN (COLE) BRUCKMAN

E35312 MISTI LANE BRUCKMAN E3531

MISTI LANE BRUCKMAN was born on 11 Nov 1974. She married MAURICE "MAURY" EDWARD BIRMINGHAM on 31 May 1997 in Walls, DeSoto Co., MS.

Children of MISTI BRUCKMAN and MAURICE BIRMINGHAM are:

i. COLBY "TAYLOR" BIRMINGHAM(E353121) was born on 15 Aug 1998 in Memphis, Shelby Co., TN.

ii. DALTON BRYANT BIRMINGHAM(E353122) was born on 26 Jan 2000 in Memphis, Shelby Co., TN.

iii. GRACI CLARE BIRMINGHAM(E353123) was born on 05 Nov 2007 in Memphis, Shelby Co., TN.

Ref: 23-Wendi Lynn Bruckman

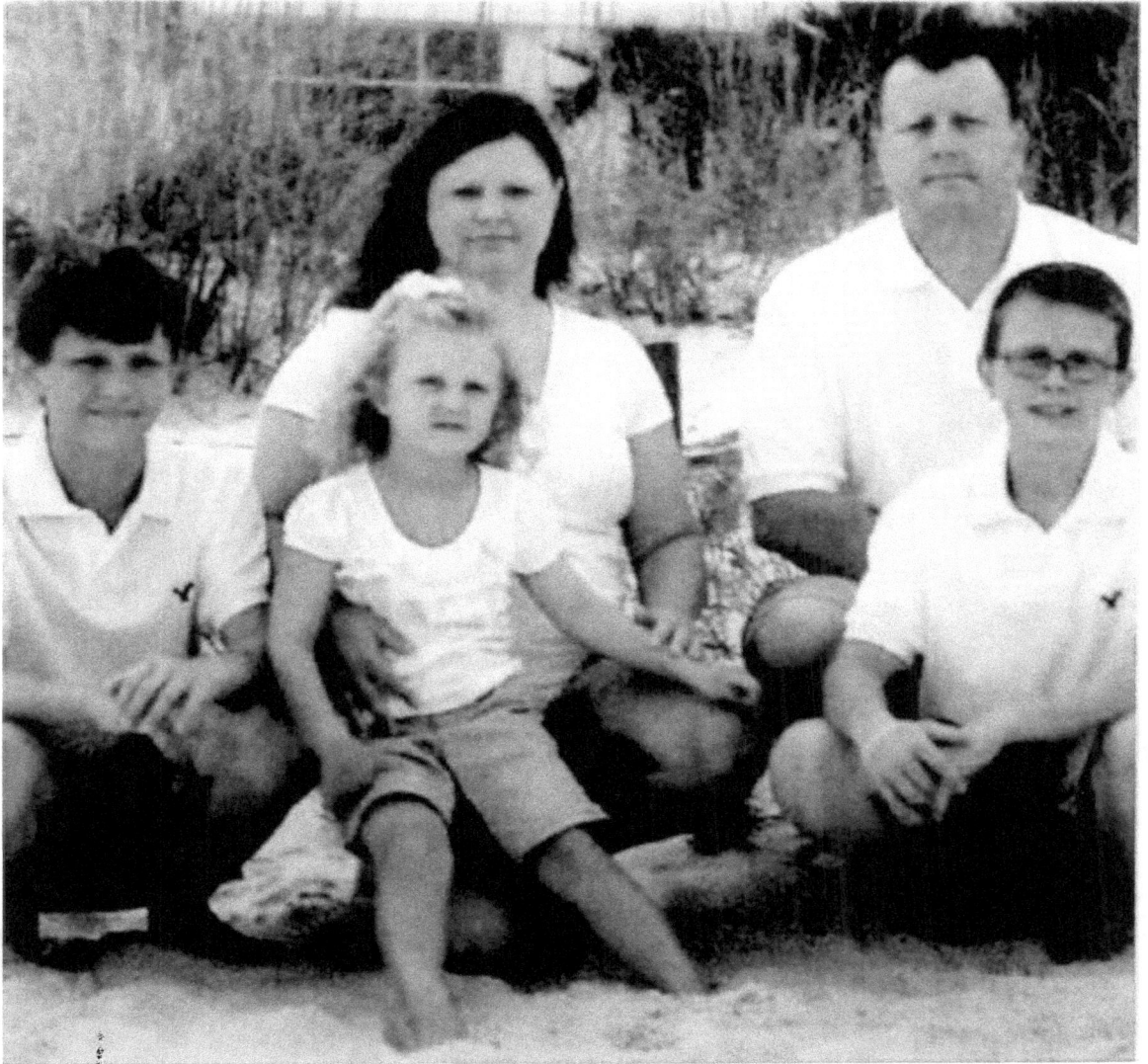

Rear: MISTI LANE (BRUCKMAN) and MAURICE EDWARD BIRMINGHAM
Front: DALTON BRYANT, GRACI CLARE, and COLBY "TAYLOR" BIRMINGHAM

E35313 WENDI LYNN BRUCKMAN E3531

WENDI LYNN BRUCKMAN was born on 26 Jan 1976. She married (1) DENNIS CLAYTON HANNAH Sr. on 02 Sep 1994 in Osceola, Mississippi Co., AR. They divorced 03 Dec 2003 in West Memphis, Crittenden Co., AR. She married (2) LANCE EDWARD PUGH on 10 Mar 2006 in Memphis, Shelby Co., TN.

Children of WENDI BRUCKMAN and DENNIS HANNAH Sr. are:

i. DENNIS "D.J." CLAYTON HANNAH Jr. (E353131) was born on 02 Feb 1997 in Memphis, Shelby Co., TN.

ii. DYLAN CHANCE HANNAH (E353132) was born on 14 Jan 1998 in Memphis, Shelby Co., TN.

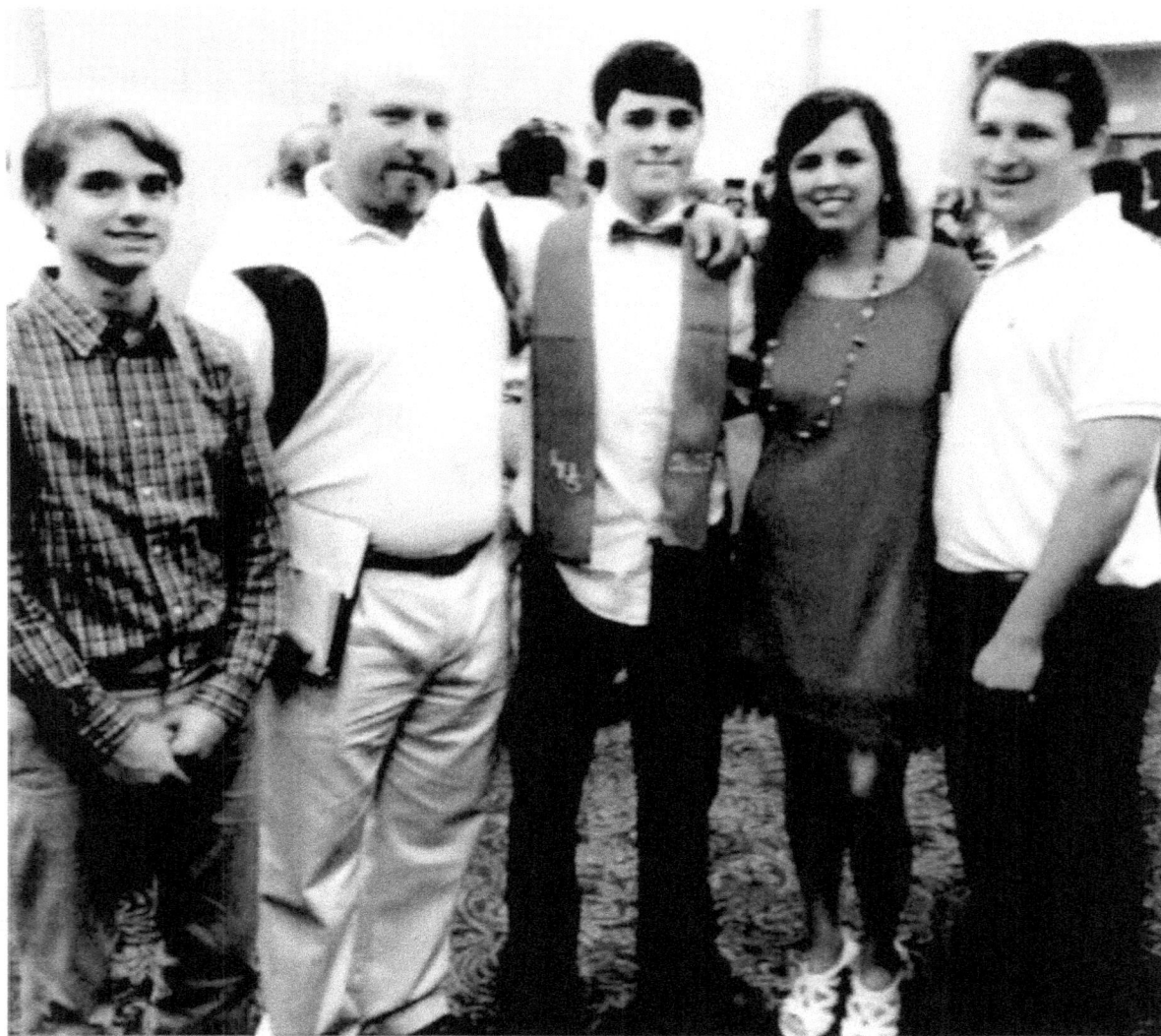

LANDON PUGH (WENDI'S STEPSON), LANCE EDWARD PUGH, DENNIS CLAYTON
HANNAH, WENDI LYNN (BRUCKMAN) PUGH, and DYLAN CHANCE HANNAH

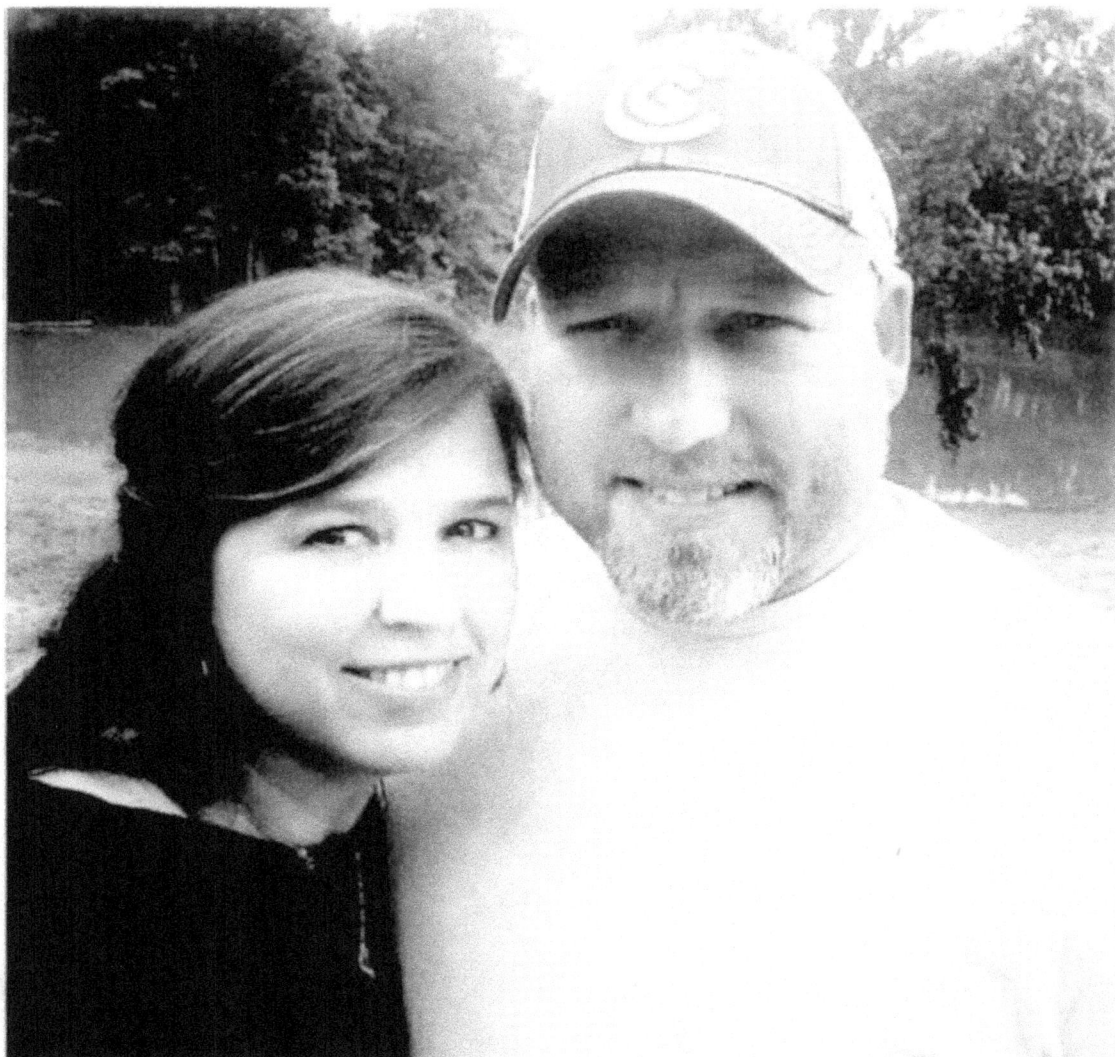

LANCE EDWARD and WENDI LYNN (BRUCKMAN) PUGH

E35314 KRISTY LEE BRUCKMAN E3531

KRISTY LEE BRUCKMAN was born on 21 Sep 1988 in Memphis, Shelby Co., TN. She married RICHARD ADAM MARSTON on 05 Jun 2010 in Oxford, Lafayette Co., MS.

Child of KRISTY BRUCKMAN and RICHARD MARSTON is:

i. CHLOE ADDISON MARSTON (E353141) was born on 26 Feb 2012 in Memphis, Shelby Co., TN.

Ref: 23-Wendi Lynn Bruckman

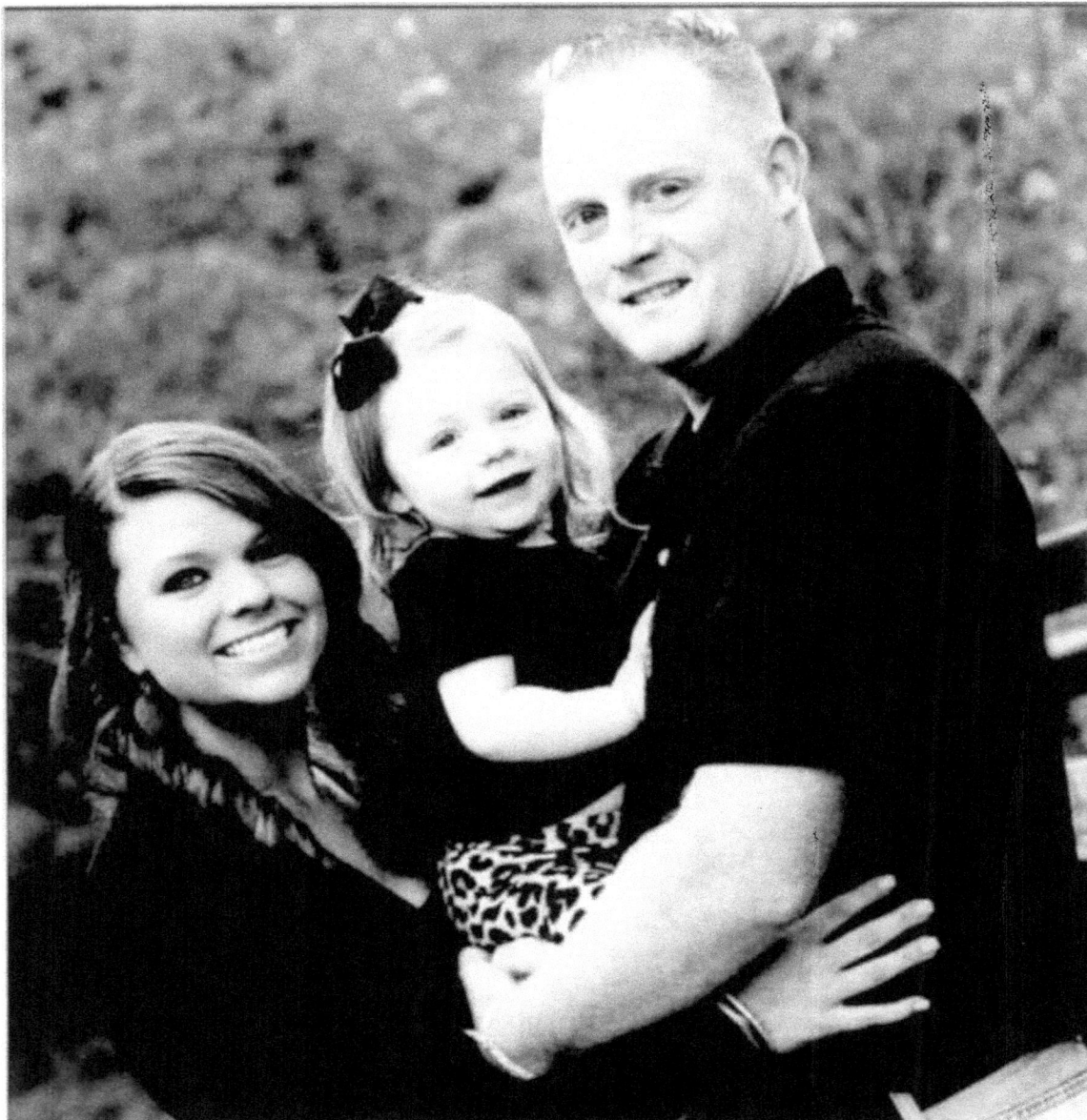

KRISTY LEE (BRUCKMAN), CHLOE ADDISON, and RICHARD ADAM MARSTON

E35321 JAMIE LOUISE BRUCKMAN E3532

JAMIE LOUISE BRUCKMAN was born on 29 Jan 1983. She married BRIAN HUGHES.

Child of JAMIE BRUCKMAN and BRIAN HUGHES is:

i. ELISHA RANDALL HUGHES (E353211) was born 6 Aug 2013, in Memphis, Shelby Co., TN.

Ref: 49, 23-Randall Eugene Bruckman

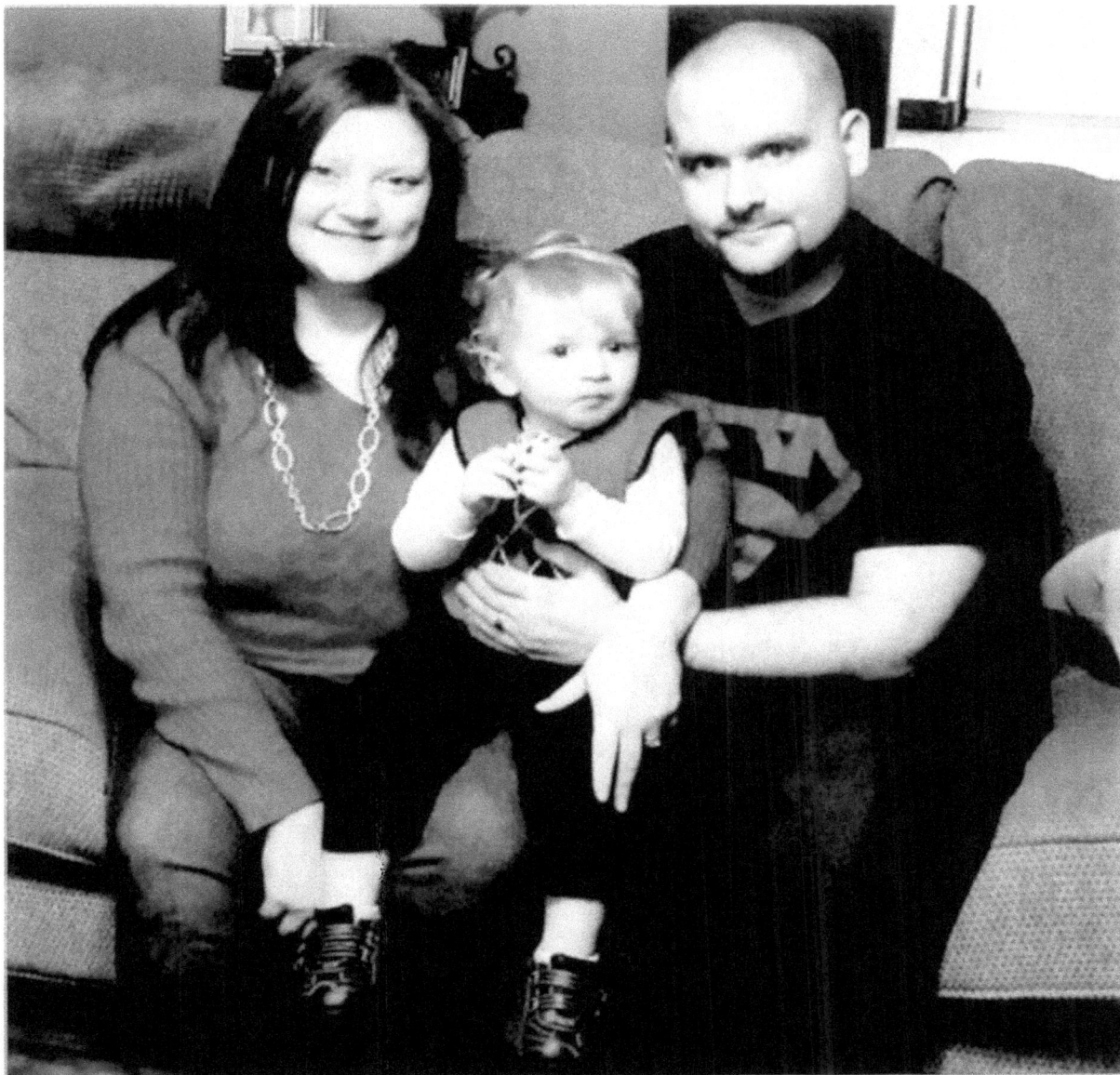

JAMIE LOUISE (BRUCKMAN) HUGHES, ELISHA "ELI" RANDALL HUGHES, BRIAN HUGHES

E35322 BAILEY ANN BRUCKMAN E3532

BAILEY ANN BRUCKMAN was born 03 May 1986. She married DAN GURLEY.

Child of BAILEY BRUCKMAN and DAN GURLEY is:

i. NICOLAS JAMES GURLEY (E353221) was born 2 Oct 2013, in Memphis, Shelby Co., TN.

Ref: 49, 23-Randall Eugene Bruckman

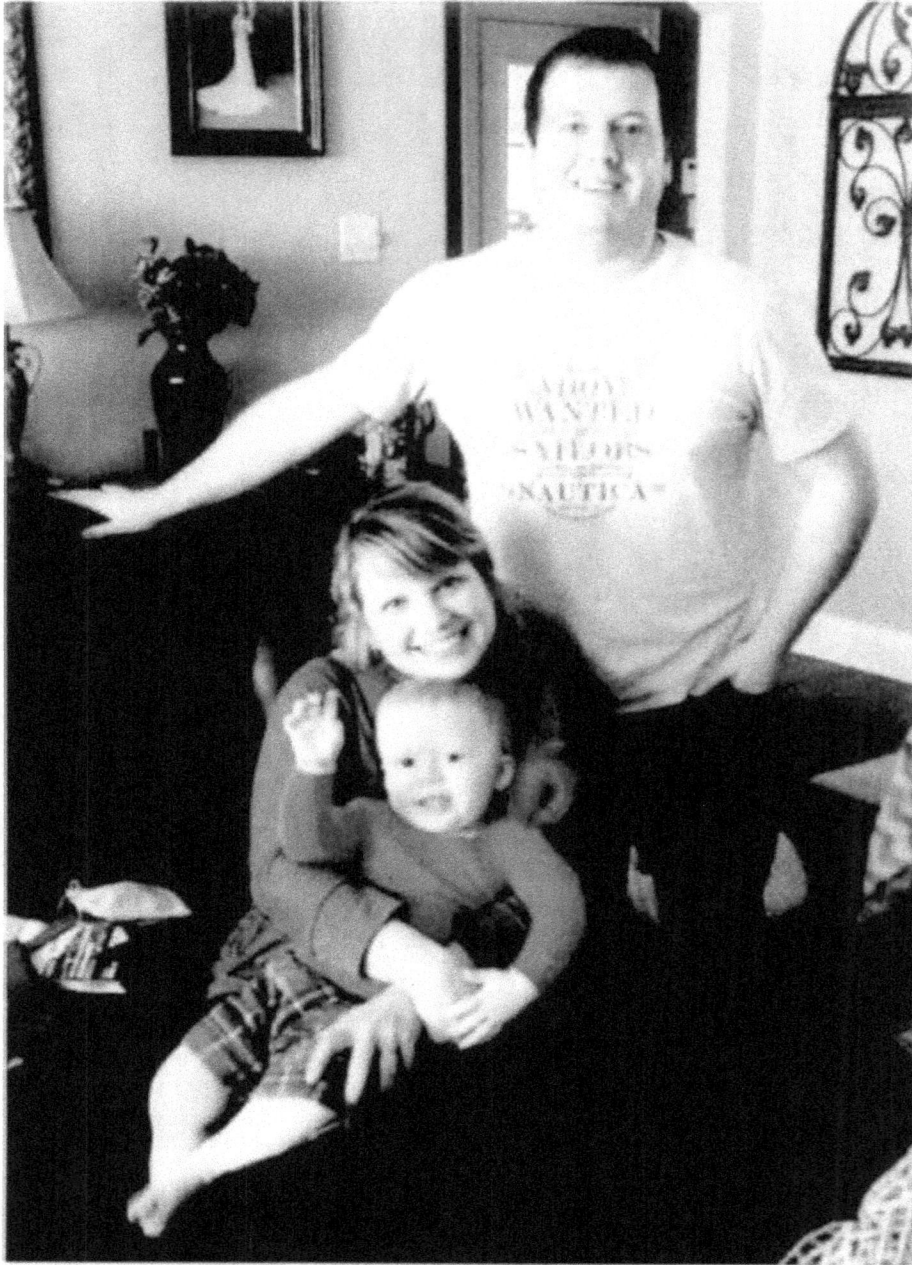

DAN GURLEY, BAILEY ANN (BRUCKMAN) GURLEY and
NICOLAS "NIC" JAMES GURLEY

E35511 YVONNE MARIE LANTZ E3551

YVONNE MARIE LANTZ was born on 18 Mar 1970 in Camp Springs, Prince George's Co., MD. She married ROBERT STEVENS.

Children of Yvonne Lantz and ROBERT STEVENS are:

i. ASHLEIGH E. STEVENS (E355111)

ii. ROBERT ANTHONY STEVENS (E355112) was born on 23 Dec 1992 in Altoona, Blair Co., PA.

Ref: 23-Yvonne Marie (Lantz) Stevens, 19

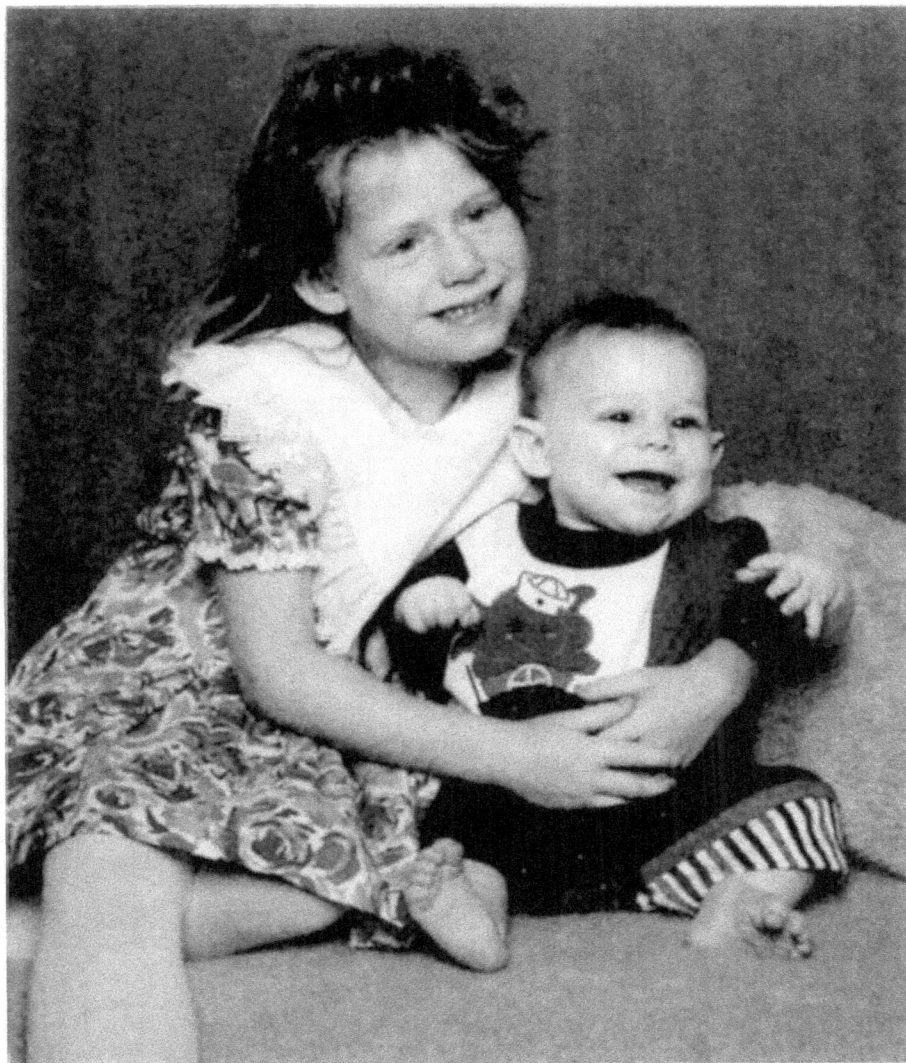

ASHLEIGH E. STEVENS and ROBERT ANTHONY STEVENS

E35512 NELSON GARFIELD LANTZ E3551

NELSON GARFIELD LANTZ was born on 25 Jun 1979 in Honolulu, HI. He married (1) SHAWN MARIE GILBERT on 10 Jan 2004 in Pensacola, Escambia Co., FL, daughter of RICHARD CONRAD GILBERT and SHEILA MARIE ROBISON. She was born 11 Jul 1977 in Birmingham, Jefferson Co., AL. They were divorced 09 Dec 1975, Pensacola, Escambia Co., FL. He married (2) RYAN SUMMER THORP, 02 Jul 2009 in Pensacola, Escambia Co., FL, daughter of KEITH EDWARD THORP and MERCEDES GAY SULLIVAN. She was born 02 Apr 1990 in St. Petersburg, Pinellas Co., FL.

Family of NELSON LANTZ and SUMMER THORP is:

i. ISABELLA ANNE MARIE BOLAR was born on 29 Dec 2007, Pensacola, Escambia Co., FL.

ii. JOCELYN ROSE LANTZ (E355121) was born on 20 Nov 2009, Pensacola, Escambia Co., FL.

Ref: 24, 25, 27-M/NGL&RST/2009ML001721 Escambia Co FL, 27-B/JRL/109-2009-109762/Escambia Co FL, 27-B/RST/109-1990-052983/Escambia Co FL,27-B/ISAMB/109-2007-249036/Escambia Co FL, 27-B/NGL/79008371/DOH HI

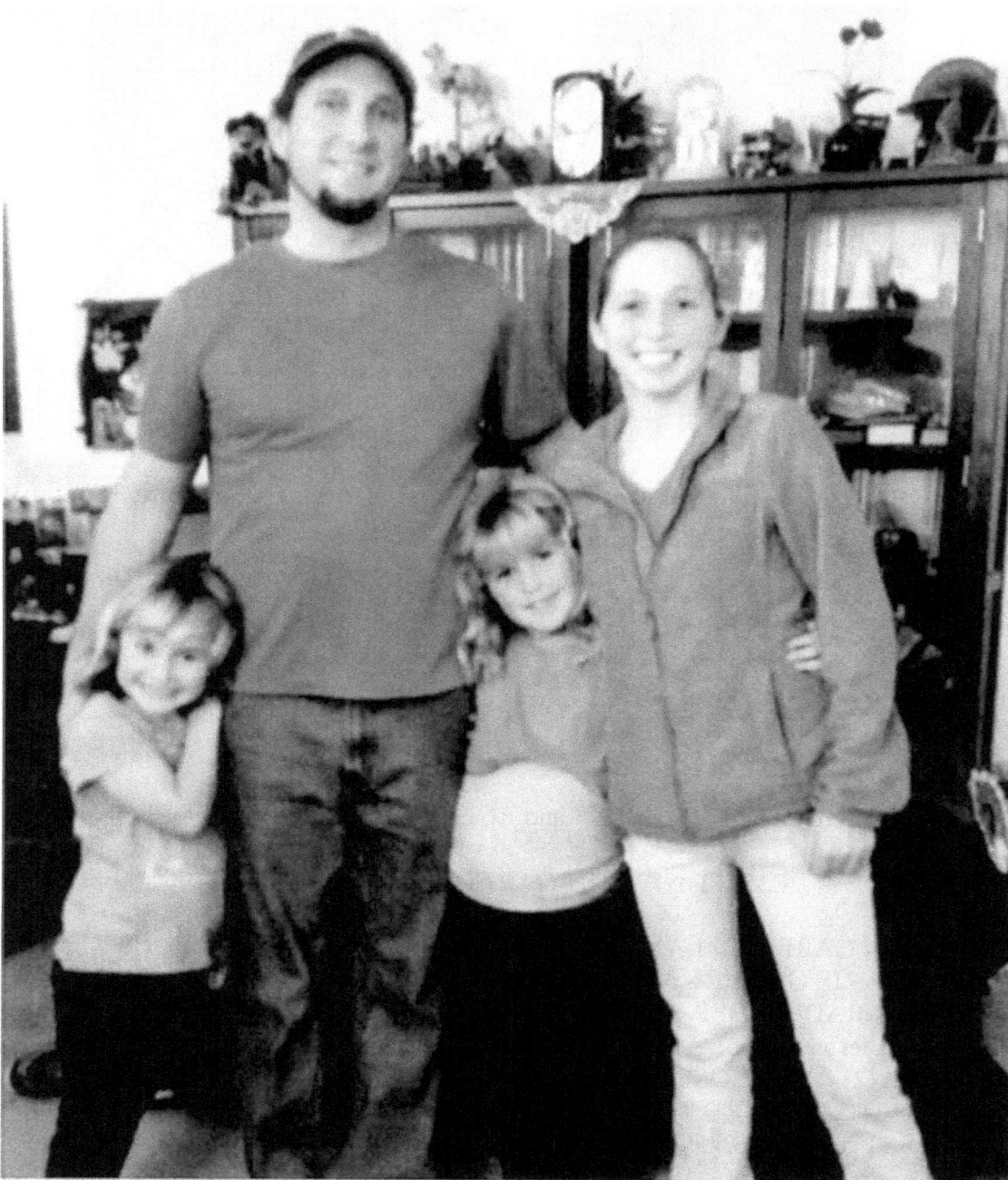

JOCELYN ROSE LANTZ, NELSON GARFIELD LANTZ, & ISABELLA ANNE MARIE BOLAR, RYAN SUMMER (THORP) LANTZ

E36221 JASON N. GRIFFITH E3622

JASON N. GRIFFITH was born on 30 Dec 1974 in WA. He married KIMBERLY ALLUISE on 12 Oct 2002 in Arlington, Snohomish Co., WA, daughter of STEPHEN and ANN MARIE (_____) ALLUISE. She was born on 03 Apr 1974 in Long Island, NY.

Children of JASON N. GRIFFITH and are:

    i. ELI GRIFFITH (E362211) was born on 05 Jan 2008 in Mt. Vernon, Skagit Co., WA.

    ii. EZRA GRIFFITH (E362212) was born on 28 Apr 2010 in Mt. Vernon, Skagit Co., WA.

Ref: 49, 23-William Richard Griffith

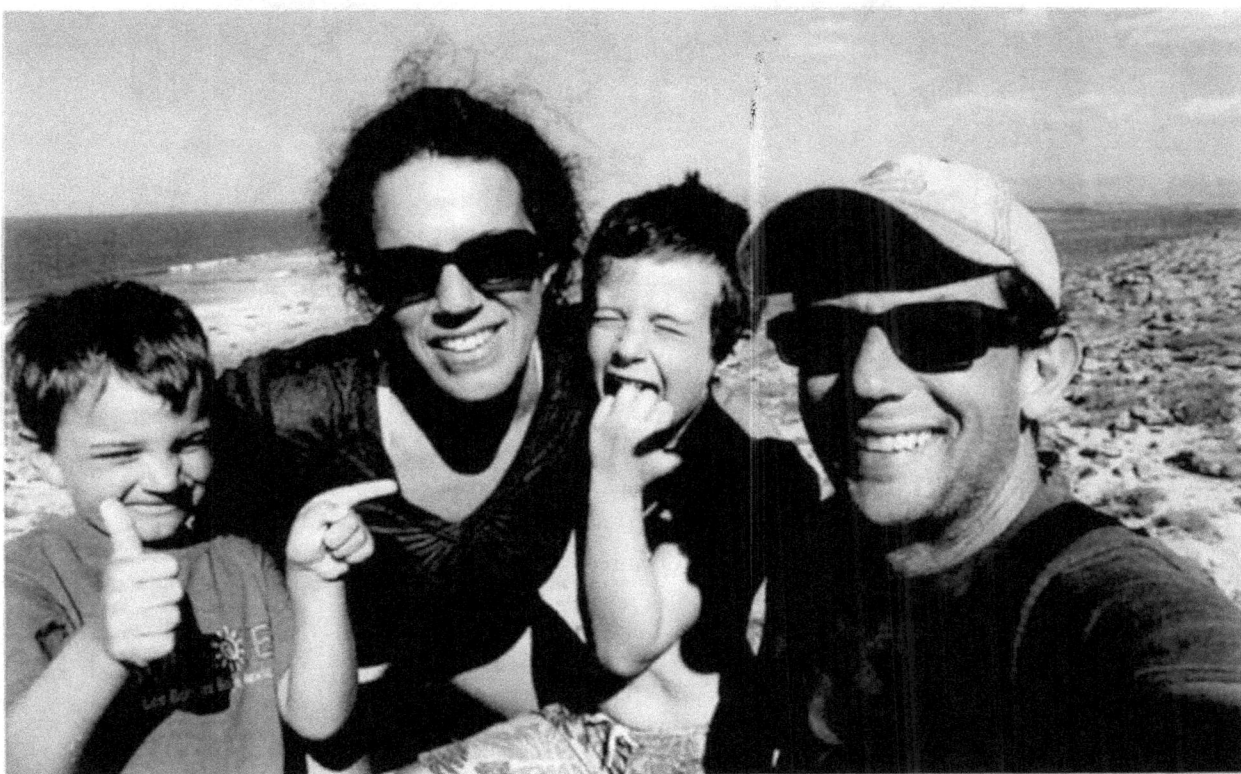

EZRA GRIFFITH, KIMBERLY A. () GRIFFITH, ELI GRIFFITH AND JASON N. GRIFFITH

E36222 ZACHARY B. GRIFFITH E3622

ZACHARY B. GRIFFITH was born on 27 Sep 1976 in Seattle, King Co., WA. He married JOY JACKSON on 21 May 2005 in Seattle, King Co., WA, daughter of JIM and EVE (_____) JACKSON. She was born on 21 Aug 1976 in Indianapolis, Marion Co., IN.

Children of ZACHARY GRIFFITH and JOY JACKSON are:

    i. CLOVER GRIFFITH (E362221) was born on 05 Aug 2008 in Seattle, King Co., WA.

ii. BARLOW GRIFFITH (E362221) was born on 23 Aug 2010 in Seattle, King Co., WA.

Ref: 49, 23-William Richard Griffith

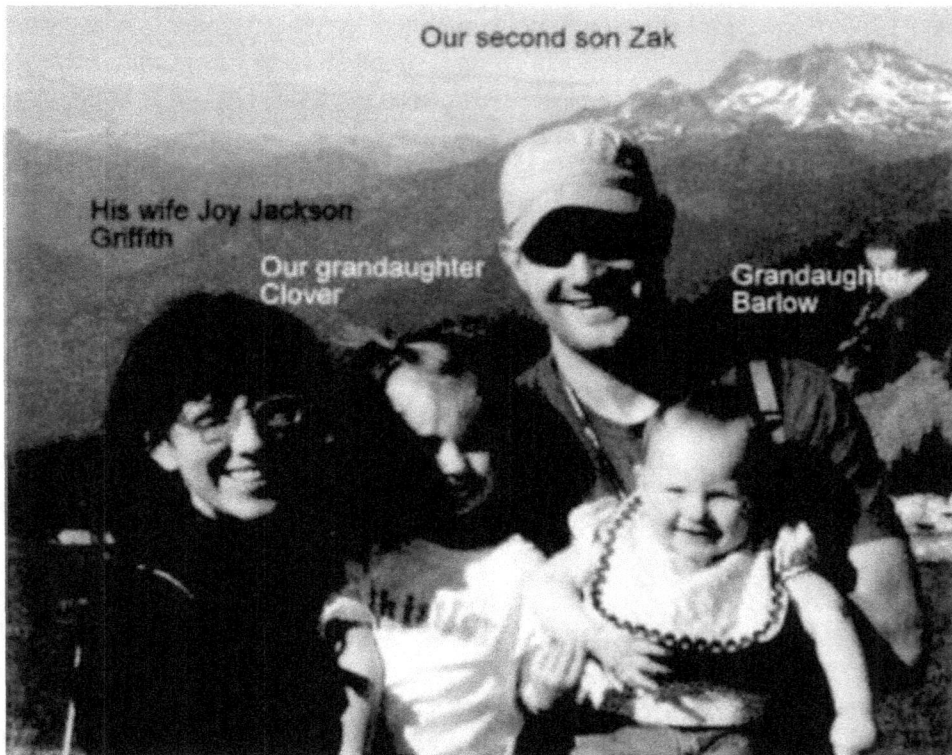

Our second son Zak

His wife Joy Jackson Griffith

Our grandaughter Clover

Grandaughter Barlow

E41231 ROBERT ALAN PETRY E4123

Dr. ROBERT ALAN PETRY married MARY LOOS.

Child of ROBERT PETRY and MARY LOOS are:

i. SKYLAR PETRY (E412311)

Ref: 26

E41232 GEORGE WILLIAM PETRY III E4123

GEORGE WILLIAM PETRY III married CAROL ALLISON in Cambria Co., PA, daughter of JOHN ALLISON.

i. MELANIE PETRY (E412321) was born on 30 Mar 1973 in Johnstown, Cambria Co., PA and died 05 May 2014 in Lorain Borough, Johnstown, Cambria Co., PA.

LORAIN BOROUGH — PETRY – Melanie F. "Mel," 41, Lorain Borough, passed away peacefully May 5, 2014, at home. Born March 30, 1973, in Johnstown. Preceded in death by grandparents, John Allison and George and Lorraine Petry. Survived by mother, Carol (Allison) Petry, and father, George Petry, both of Lorain Borough; sister, Dawn, married to Keith Null, Ferndale; loving fiancee of 20 years, Robert Owens, Lorain Borough;

grandmother, Helen Larnek, Johnstown; cherished niece, Allyson Null; numerous aunts and uncles; and loving cat, Angel. Melanie was an active supporter of the Penn Drop In Center, and went to culinary arts school at Hiram G. Andrews where she met Bob. She was a gentle, loving person who will be missed by her family and friends. Family will receive friends from 2 to 4 and 6 until celebration of life at 8 p.m. Wednesday, May 7, at Moskal & Kennedy Colonial Funeral Home, Pastor Robert R. Wagner, officiating. Interment, Forest Lawn Cemetery.
(www.moskalandkennedyfuneralhome.com/obituaries/obit%20files/melanie.petry.html)

    ii. DAWN PETRY (E412322)

Ref: 42

E42621 STACY LUDY E4262

STACY LUDY married _____ BRUNING.

Children of STACY LUDY and _____ BRUNING are:

    i. ARIN BRUNING (E426211)

    ii. SARA BRUNING (E426212)

Ref: 44

E42111 CHRISTOPHER F. COWAN E4211

CHRISTOPHER F. COWAN was born on 12 Oct 1950 in PA. He married ANNE CARRIGG.

Children of CHRISTOPHER COWAN and ANNE CARRIGG are:

    i. CLAIRE ELAINE COWAN (E421111)

    ii. MARY ROSE COWAN (E421112) married _____ KROGER

    iii. CHRISTOPHER LOYAL COWAN (E421113)

Ref: 49

E42112 SUSAN COWAN E4211

SUSAN COWAN married JAMES W. JOHNSTON.

Children of SUSAN COWAN and JAMES JOHNSTON are:

    i. JENNIE JOHNSTON (E421121)

    ii. JEFF JOHNSTON (E421122)

iii. DOUG JOHNSTON (E421123)

Ref:

E42113 CHARLOTTE COWAN E4211

CHARLOTTE COWAN was born on 01 Oct 1956. She married ERSKINE FULCHER. He was born on 10 Aug 1956.

Child of CHARLOTTE COWAN and ERSKINE ODEN FULCHER is:

i. ERIC J. FULCHER (E421131)

ii. EMILIE FULCHER (E421132)

Ref: 49

E42114 CURTIS C. COWAN E4211

CURTIS C. COWAN was born on He married MONICA DUNBAR. She was born on 09 Nov 1962.

Children of CURTIS COWAN and MONICA DUNBAR are:

i. ERIC HAURY COWAN (E421141)

ii. ALLISON COWAN (E421142)

iii. LISA CLAIR COWAN (E421143)

Ref: 49

E42211 DARLENE L. GIFFIN E4221

DARLENE L. GIFFIN married LARRY BENSHOFF in PA.

i. BRIAN BENSHOFF (E422111)

ii. JEFFREY BENSHOFF (E422112)

Ref: 44

E42212 MILTON BARRY GIFFIN E4221

MILTON BARRY GIFFIN married DIANA "DEE" UNGER.

i. ERIC GIFFIN (E422121)

Ref: 44

E42231 R. LYNN WEIGLE E4223

R. LYNN WEIGLE married ESTHER MOSTOLLER.

Child of R. WEIGLE and ESTHER MOSTOLLER is:

i. JEREMY LYNN WEIGLE (E422311)

Ref: 44

E42313 DONNA L. HARTMAN E4231

DONNA L. HARTMAN was born on 16 Dec 1955 in PA. She married ROBERT J. PLESS. He was born on 15 Sep 1956.

Child of DONNA HARTMAN and ROBERT PLESS is:

i. CAROL PLESS (E423131) was born in NJ.

Ref: 49

E42542 KAREN E. FUREDY E4254

KAREN E. FUREDY was born on 16 Oct 1968 in PA. She married MICHAEL VEITH.

Children of KAREN FUREDY and MICHAEL VEITH are:

i. RYAN VEITH (E425421)

ii. KAYLA VEITH (E425422)

iii. BROOKE VEITH (E425423)

Ref: 49

E42741 THOMAS LEROY WINEBRENNER II E4274

THOMAS LEROY WINEBRENNER II

Children of THOMAS WINEBRENNER and _____ are:

i. SEAN THOMAS WINEBRENNER (E427411)

ii. DYLAN PATRICK WINEBRENNER (E427412)

Ref: 49

E48213 RHONDA MICHELLE MULL E4821

RHONDA MICHELLE MULL married RICK DADDIO.

Children of RHONDA MULL and RICK DADDIO are:

   i. RICKY DADDIO (E482131)

   ii. RYANN DADDIO (E482132)

   iii. RYLEE DADDIO (E482133)

Ref: 44

E48433 CHANTAY ELIZABETH MULL E4843

CHANTAY ELIZABETH MULL married MICHAEL LAWSON.

Children of CHANTAY MULL and MICHAEL LAWSON are:

   i. CATHARINE LAWSON (E484331)

   ii. ROBERT LAWSON (E484332)

Ref: 44

E48434 TONYA YVONNE MULL E4843

TONYA YVONNE MULL She married KENNETH CHRISTNER Jr.

Children of TONYA MULL and KENNETH CHRISTNER Jr. are:

   i. KENNETH CHRISTNER III (E484341)

   ii. TIFFANI CHRISTNER (E484342)

   iii. TORI CHRISTNER (E484343)

   iv. TRINITI CHRISTNER (E484344)

   v. TIANI CHRISTNER (E484345)

Ref: 44

E355111 ASHLEIGH E. STEVENS E35511

ASHLEIGH E. STEVENS was born on 01 Sep 1987 in Altoona, Blair Co., PA.

Child of ASHLEIGH STEVENS and _____ is:

i. JASIAH EDWARD STEVENS (E3551111) was born in 2005 in Altoona, Blair Co., PA.

Ref: 23-Yvonne Marie (Lantz) Stevens, 19

E412322 DAWN PETRY E41232

DAWN PETRY married KEITH NULL.

Child of DAWN PETRY and KEITH NULL is.

i. ALLYSON RAE NULL (E4123221)

Ref: 26, 44

E421131 ERIC J. FULCHER E42113

ERIC J. FULCHER was born 22 Feb 1982.

Child of ERIC FULCHER is:

i. ERIC J. FULCHER Jr. (E4211311)

Ref: 49

REFERENCES

1. *Somerset County Naturalizations Records*: Somerset County Courthouse, 111 East Union Street, Somerset, PA 15501.

2. Robertta E. & Thomas C. Imler. Bedford County Pennsylvania Cemeteries. (1975).

3. Floyd G. Hoenstine. *The 1955 Year Book of the Pennsylvania Society Sons of the American Revolution.* (Pittsburgh, PA: PASSAR, 1956)

4. Ancestry.com. *1850 United States Federal Census* [database on-line]. (Provo, UT, USA: Ancestry.com Operations, Inc., 2009). Images reproduced by FamilySearch.

5. Ancestry.com. *1860 United States Federal Census* [database on-line]. (Provo, UT, USA: Ancestry.com Operations, Inc., 2009). Images reproduced by FamilySearch.

6. Ancestry.com. *1870 United States Federal Census* [database on-line]. (Provo, UT, USA: Ancestry.com Operations, Inc., 2009). Images reproduced by FamilySearch.

7. Ancestry.com and The Church of Jesus Christ of Latter-day Saints. *1880 United States FederalCensus* [database on-line]. (Provo, UT, USA: Ancestry.com Operations Inc, 2010).

8. Ancestry.com. *1900 United States Federal Census* [database on-line]. (Provo, UT, USA: Ancestry.com Operations Inc, 2004).

9. Ancestry.com. *1910 United States Federal Census* [database on-line]. (Provo, UT, USA: Ancestry.com Operations Inc, 2006).

10. Ancestry.com. *1920 United States Federal Census* [database on-line]. (Provo, UT, USA: Ancestry.com Operations Inc, 2010). Images reproduced by FamilySearch.

11. Ancestry.com. *1930 United States Federal Census* [database on-line]. Provo, UT, USA: Ancestry.com Operations Inc, 2002.

12. Ancestry.com. *1940 United States Federal Census* [database on-line]. (Provo, UT, USA: Ancestry.com Operations, Inc., 2012).

13. Ancestry.com. *U.S. City Directories, 1821-1989* [database on-line]. Provo, UT, USA: Ancestry.com Operations, Inc., 2011.

14. Linda Shillinger. *The Genealogy of the Keller Family.* (Hollidaysburg, PA: Blair County Genealogical Society, 2006).

15. Ancestry.com. *New York, State Census, 1825-1925* [database on-line]. Provo, UT, USA: Ancestry.com Operations, Inc., 2012.

16. *Henry Dilling Detwiler Bible* in possession of Daniel Bruckman, Altoona, Blair Co., PA, 1985

17. Thomas Capek. *The Cech (Bohemian) Community of New York with Introductory Remarks on "The Cechoslovaks in the United States".* (New York: The Czechoslovak section of America's making, Inc., 1921).

18. Hyman B. Grinstein. *The Rise of the Jewish Community of New York 1654-1860.* (Philadelphia: The Jewish Publication Society of America, 1945).

19. Raymond C. Lantz. *Descendants of Johann Jacob Lantz 1721-1789 Immigrant Settler of*

Albany Township, Berks County, Pennsylvania. (Berwyn Heights, MD: Heritage Books, Inc., 2013).

20.   Isidore Singer & Cyrus Adler, (Eds.). The Jewish Encyclopedia: *A Descriptive Record of the History, Religion, Literature, and Customs of the Jewish People from the Earliest Times to the Present Day, Volume 3.* (New York: KTAV, 1964).

21.   Department of Commerce and Labor, Bureau of the Census. *Official Register of the United States, Containing a List of the Officers and Employees in the Civil, Military, and Naval Service.* Digitized books (77 volumes). Oregon State Library, Salem, Oregon. (Washington, DC: GPO, 1883).

22.   Czech Republic National Archives. *Registers of Jewish Religious Communities in the Czech regions (1735) 1784 – 1949 (1960),* [database on-line with Images]. (Prague: www.Badatelna.eu, 2014)

23.   *Named descendant/researcher* provided data and/or remarks.

24.   Raymond C. Lantz. *Lantz-Crossley an Experience in Genealogy: Volume I, A-E, 2nd Edition* (Westminster, MD: Heritage Books, Inc., 2009).

25.   Raymond C. Lantz. *Lantz-Crossley an Experience in Genealogy: Supplement I to Volumes I-IV, 2ndEdition* (Westminster, MD: Heritage Books, Inc., 2011).

26.   Find A Grave, Inc. *Find A Grave.* [database on-line] (www.findagrave.com, 2012).

27.   State & County Vital Records: *Birth (B), Death (D) or Marriage (M) records.* Type record/name(s) or initials of individual(s)/file, certificate number or book and page/location of record office in where filed, or repository in which copy was found - e.g. archives.

28.   *Territorial Enterprise Marriage Notices (Virginia City, Nevada), 1866-67* [database on-line]. Web site: genealogytrails.com/nev/storey/marr/virgcitymarrnotes.html (2014).

29.   Dodd, Jordan, Liahona Research, Comp. *Colorado Marriages, 1859-1900* [database on-line]. Provo, UT, USA: Ancestry.com Operations Inc, 2000.

30.   Ancestry.com. *Colorado, Statewide Marriage Index, 1900-1939* [database on-line]. Provo, UT, USA: Ancestry.com Operations, Inc., 2014.

31.   Familysearch.org. *Colorado Statewide Marriage Index, 1853-2006.* (https://familysearch.org/pal:/MM9.1.1/KNQ5-6KT).

32.   Familysearch.org. *New York, State Census, 1855.* (https://familysearch.org/pal:/MM9.1.1/K67X-8JZ)

33.   Ancestry.com. *California, Death Index, 1940-1997* [database on-line]. Provo, UT, USA: Ancestry.com Operations Inc, 2000.

34.   Standford University. *Alumni Directory and Ten-Year Book Graduates and Non-Graduates III 1891-1920.* (California: Standford University, 1921).

35.   Familysearch.org. *California, County Marriages, 1850-1952.* (https://familysearch.org/pal:/MM9.1.1/KZ3X-KBZ).

36.   Waterman, Watkins & Co. *History of Bedford, Somerset and Fulton Counties Pennsylvania.* (Chicago: Waterman, Watkins & Co., 1884).

37. Familysearch.org. *New York, Births and Christenings, 1640-1962.* (https://familysearch.org/pal:/MM9.1.1/FDYM-GFH).

38. Familysearch.org. *New York, Marriages, 1686-1980.* (https://familysearch.org/pal:/MM9.1.1/F6H8-LM2)

39. Ancestry.com. *U.S. Passport Applications, 1795-1925* [database on-line]. (Provo, UT, USA: Ancestry.com Operations, Inc., 2007).

40. Ancestry.com. *New York, New York, Death Index, 1862-1948* [database on-line]. (Provo, UT, USA: Ancestry.com Operations, Inc., 2014).

41. Ancestry.com. *British Columbia Marriage Registrations, 1859-1932.* (https://familysearch.org/pal:/MM9.1.1/JD87-NK2).

42. Ancestry.com. *U.S., Social Security Death Index, 1935-2014* [database on-line]. (Provo, UT, USA: Ancestry.com Operations Inc, 2011).

43. Familysearch.org. *Michigan, Deaths and Burials, 1800-1995.* (https://familysearch.org/pal:/MM9.1.1/FH3F-TVN)

44. USGenWeb Archives. *Somerset County, PA Obits.* (http://usgwarchives.net/pa/somerset/obits/)

45. Ancestry.com. *Historical Data Systems, comp. U.S., Civil War Soldier Records and Profiles, 1861-1865* [database on-line]. (Provo, UT, USA: Ancestry.com Operations Inc, 2009).

46. Ancestry.com. *National Archives and Records Administration. U.S., Civil War Pension Index: General Index to Pension Files, 1861-1934* [database on-line]. (Provo, UT, USA: Ancestry.com Operations Inc, 2000).

47. Ancestry.com. *Pennsylvania, Veteran Compensation Applications, WWII, 1950* [database on-line]. (Provo, UT, USA: Ancestry.com Operations, Inc., 2013).

48. Ancestry.com. *National Archives and Records Administration. U.S. World War II Army Enlistment Records, 1938-1946* [database on-line]. (Provo, UT, USA: Ancestry.com Operations Inc, 2005).

49. Familysearch.org. *United States Public Records, 1970-2009.* (https://familysearch.org/pal:/MM9.1.1/QJJD-SPJZ)

50. Familysearch.org. *Florida, Death Index, 1877-1998.* (https://familysearch.org/pal:/MM9.1.1/VVWM-SWG)

51. Ancestry.com. *Washington, Select Death Certificates, 1907-1960* [database on-line]. (Provo, UT, USA: Ancestry.com Operations, Inc., 2014).

52. Ancestry.com. *United States Obituary Collection* [database on-line]. (Provo, UT, USA: Ancestry.com Operations Inc, 2006).

53. Ancestry.com. *Washington Death Index, 1940-1996* [database on-line]. (Provo, UT, USA: Ancestry.com Operations Inc, 2002).

54. Familysearch.org. *Pennsylvania, County Marriages, 1885-1950.* (https://familysearch.org/pal:/MM9.1.1/VFSK-BY3).

55. Familysearch.org. *California, County Birth and Death Records, 1800-1994.* (https://familysearch.org/pal:/MM9.1.1/QV37-6KMB).

56. Familysearch.org. *Idaho, Death Certificates, 1911-1937.* (https://familysearch.org/pal:/MM9.1.1/FLT1-HXR).

57. Wikipedia contributors. *Wikipedia, The Free Encyclopedia.* (http://en.wikipedia.org/wiki/).

58. Kathleen Edwards Small & J. Larry Smith. *History of Tulare County and Kings County, California.* (Chicago: The S. J. Clarke Publishing Company, 1926).

59. Ancestry.com. *Ohio Department of Health. Ohio, Deaths, 1908-1932, 1938-2007* [database on-line]. (Provo, UT, USA: Ancestry.com Operations Inc, 2010).

60. Jewish Heritage Europe, 2014. *Czech Republic: Restored synagogue in Loštice dedicated.* (http://www.jewish-heritage-europe.eu/2014/10/08/czech-republic-restored-synagogue-in-lostice-dedicated/%E2%80%9D).

61. E. Randol Schoenberg & Julius Mueller, 2013. *Getting Started With Czech-Jewish Genealogy.* (http://www.jewishgen.org/AustriaCzech/czechguide.html).

62. Jewfaq.com. *Judaism 101: Jewish Surnames.* (http://www.jewfaq.org/jnames.htm)

63. International Association of Jewish Genealogical Societies, 2014. *International Jewish Cemetery Project Lostice: Sumperk, Moravia.* (http://www.iajgsjewishcemeteryproject.org/czech-republic/lostice.html)

64. Respect and Tolerance. *Lostice: History of Jewish Community.* (http://archiv.respectandtolerance.com/en/lostice/216-lostice-history-of-jewish-community.html)

65. Geni.com. *Jewish Families from Kroměříž (Kremsier), Moravia, Czech Republic.* (http://www.geni.com/projects/Jewish-Families-from-Kromeriz-Kremsier-Moravia-Czech-Republic/13164).

66. Geni.com. *Jewish Families from Loštice (Loschitz), Moravia, Czech Republic.* (http://www.geni.com/projects/Jewish-Families-from-Lo%C5%A1tice-Loschitz-Moravia-Czech-Republic/13136).

67. Raymond C. Lantz. *Dr. Jacob George Bruckman (1800-1885) Truths and Myths about a 19th Century German Immigrant Doctor?* ("Blair County Genealogical Society Newsletter", March April May 2010 Issue, Volume 31 Number 1, p. 4-6)

68. Raymond C. Lantz. *Dr. Jacob George Bruckman (1800-1885) Truths and Myths about a 19th Century German Jewish Immigrant Doctor Continued...* ("Blair County Genealogical Society Newsletter", September, October, November 2010 Issue, Volume 34 Number 3, p. 18-24)

69. Adam Mendelsohn. *Bruckman, Henrietta.* Encyclopedia Judaica 2nd ed., Vol. 4, p. 220. (Jerusalem: Keter Publishing House, LTD., 2007).

70. Jacob Rader Marcus. *United States Jewry, 1776-1985.* (Detroit, MI: Wayne State University Press, 1993). Vol. 3, p. 66.

71. Miloslav Rechcigl, Jr. *Czech American Timeline Chronology of Milestones in the History of Czechs in America.* (Bloomington, IN: AuthorHouse, 2013). p. 46, 48, 53 & 56

72. Thomas Capek. *The Čech (Bohemian) Community in New York.* (New York:

Czechoslovak Section of America's Making, 1921). p. 60

73. Alexander Bruckman, book HBMa No.1557 stored in National Archives of Prague, on the page 12 – image 15, Registers of Jewish Religious Communities in the Czech regions, The National Archives, (1735) 1784 - 1949 (1960). (http://www.badatelna.eu/reprodukce/ ?fondId= 1073&zaznamId=1108115&reproId=3728793)

74. Familysearch.org. Tennessee, State Marriage Index, 1780-2002. (https://familysearch .org/pal:/MM9.1.1/VNZZ-VQZ)

75. Familysearch.org. New York, State Census, 1905. (https://familysearch.org/pal:/ MM9.1.1/SPNH-F22)

76. Ancestry.com. *West Virginia, Births Index, 1853-1969* [database on-line]. (Provo, UT, USA: Ancestry.com Operations, Inc., 2011.)

77. Ancestry.com. *California, Marriage Index, 1960-1985* [database on-line]. (Provo, UT, USA: Ancestry.com Operations Inc, 2007.)

78. Ancestry.com. *California, Divorce Index, 1966-1984* [database on-line]. (Provo, UT, USA: Ancestry.com Operations Inc, 2007.)

Africa
  Shirley Mae
    95
Allison
  Carol
    150
Allmond
  Rowena A.
    77
Alluise
  Kimberly
    149
  Stephen
    149
Avery
  Marvin E.
    88
  Mary Authalia
    88, 89
Badaracco
  Joseph
    115
  Karen M.
    115
Bailey
  John Alva
    119
  Marcella Lillian
    63, 67
  Pamela Denise
    119, 120
Barnard
  Steve
    94
Barron
  Judy
    111
Beasom
  Garrett A.
    81
  Herman
    61
  Jeffrey A.
    81
  Kenneth Bishop
    61
  Kenneth Girard

    61, 81
  Michael E.
    81
  Samantha G.
    81
  Thelma A.
    61
Bender
  Fred
    108
Benrimo
  Dona
    20
Benshoff
  Brian
    152
  Jeffrey
    152
  Larry
    152
Benson
  Mr.
    103
Berkdale
  Ruth
    108
Berkheimer
  Amy Renee
    130
Birmingham
  Colby
    140, 141
  Dalton Bryant
    140, 141
  Graci Clare
    140, 141
  Maurice Edward
    140, 141
  Maury
    140
  Taylor
    140, 141
Bolar
  Isabella Anne
    148
Borror
  Mr.

    79
Bowman
  Anna
    111
Brooks
  Charles Duane
    115, 116, 117
  Peter Vernon
    115
  Rachel Louise
    116
  Rebecca Ann
    116
  Ruth Amber
    116
Brown
  Charles William
    83
  Josephine Louise
    66, 83, 84
Bruckman
  Albert
    19
  Alexander
    3, 12, 22
  Alice May
    46, 61
  Aloys
    12, 20
  Anna Elizabeth
    46, 58
  Arnold
    80
  Arthur
    20
  Arthur Franklin
    46, 68
  Bailey Ann
    119, 145
  Barbara
    80
  Bettina
    23
  Beverly A.
    97
  Brad
    139

163

Heritage Books by Raymond C. Lantz:

Ancestors, Descendants and Allied Lines of Dr. Jacob George Bruckman, 1800–1885, and Dr. Philip Bruckman, 1797–1874, German Jewish Immigrant Physicians and Brothers from Böhmen, Austria (Now Czech Republic)

Bureau of Indian Affairs: Special Agent Horace B. Durant's 1907 Durant Roll Field Notes; Correspondence and Field Notes Relating to the Census Roll of All Members or Descendants of Members Who Were on the Roll of the Ottawa and the Chippewa Tribes of Michigan in 1870, and Living on March 4, 1907

Descendants of Johann Jacob Lantz, 1721–1789, Immigrant Settler of Albany Township, Berks County, Pennsylvania

Descendants of Johann Jacob Lantz, 1721–1789, Immigrant Settler of Albany Township, Berks County, Pennsylvania Supplement I

Lantz-Crossley: An Experience in Genealogy

Lantz-Crossley: An Experience in Genealogy, Volume I, A–E, Second Edition

Lantz-Crossley: An Experience in Genealogy, Volume II, F–J, Second Edition

Lantz-Crossley: An Experience in Genealogy, Volume III, K–O, Second Edition

Lantz-Crossley: An Experience in Genealogy, Volume IV, P–Z, Second Edition

Lantz-Crossley: An Experience in Genealogy, Supplement I to Volumes I–IV, Second Edition

Lantz-Crossley: An Experience in Genealogy, Supplement II to Volumes I–IV, Second Edition

Ottawa and Chippewa Indians of Michigan, 1855–1868

Ottawa and Chippewa Indians of Michigan, 1870–1909

Potawatomi Indians of Michigan, 1843–1904 Including Some Ottawa and Chippewa, 1843–1866 and Potawatomi of Indiana, 1869 and 1885

Seminole Indians of Florida: 1850–1874

Seminole Indians of Florida: 1875–1879

www.ingramcontent.com/pod-product-compliance
Lightning Source LLC
Chambersburg PA
CBHW080612270326
41928CB00016B/3029